New technology always raises compelling ethical questions. As those in medicine increasingly depend on computers and other intelligent machines, the intersection of ethics, computing, and the health professions grows more complex and significant.

This book identifies and addresses the full range of ethical issues that arise when intelligent machines are used in medicine, nursing, psychology, and allied health professions. It maps and explores a variety of important issues and controversies, including ethics and evaluation in computational medicine, patient and provider confidentiality, and responsibility for the use of computers in medicine. The expert contributors suggest real and practical approaches to difficult problems, such as the appropriate use of decision-support systems, outcomes research and computational prognosis, including mortality predictions, and computer-based biomedical research, especially meta-analysis.

As the first systematic survey of the field, this book is appropriate for students, researchers, and health care professionals. It will be welcomed particularly by participants in bioethics and medical informatics, and also by physicians, nurses, and those in health administration and medicolegal work.

ETHICS, COMPUTING, AND MEDICINE

ETHICS, COMPUTING, AND MEDICINE

Informatics and the transformation of health care

Edited by

KENNETH W. GOODMAN

Director, Forum for Bioethics and Philosophy
University of Miami

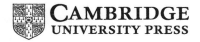
CAMBRIDGE
UNIVERSITY PRESS

PUBLISHED BY THE PRESS SYNDICATE OF THE UNIVERSITY OF CAMBRIDGE
The Pitt Building, Trumpington Street, Cambridge, United Kingdom

CAMBRIDGE UNIVERSITY PRESS
The Edinburgh Building, Cambridge CB2 2RU, United Kingdom
40 West 20th Street, New York, NY 10011-4211,USA
10 Stamford Road, Oakleigh, Melbourne 3166, Australia

First published 1998
Reprinted 1999

Printed in the United States of America

Typeset in Times Roman

Library of Congress Cataloging-in-Publication Data
Ethics, computing, and medicine : informatics and the transformation
of health care / edited by Kenneth W. Goodman.

p. cm.

Includes index.

ISBN 0-521-46486-2 (hardbound). ISBN 0-521-46905-8 (pbk.)
1. Medicine – Data processing – Moral and ethical aspects.
I. Goodman, Kenneth W., 1954–   .
R858.E84   1998
174'.2 – dc21   97–10265
                                                                         CIP

A catalog record for this book is available from
the British Library

ISBN 0 521 46486 2 hardback
ISBN 0 521 46905 8 paperback

Contents

Preface

From the outset, the idea was to try to draw together parts of three vast areas of inquiry – ethics, computing, and medicine – and produce a document that would be accessible by and useful to scholars and practitioners in each domain. Daunting projects are made possible by supportive institutions and colleagues. Fortunately in this case, the support exceeded the daunt.

The idea for the book came while I was at Carnegie Mellon University's Center for Machine Translation and Center for the Advancement of Applied Ethics, and the University of Pittsburgh's Center for Medical Ethics. These three centers of excellence fostered a congenial and supportive environment in which to launch a novel project. Deep thanks are due Jaime Carbonell, Preston Covey, Peter Madsen, Alan Meisel, and Sergei Nirenburg.

In 1992 I organized a session on "Computers and Ethics in Medicine" at the annual meeting of the American Association for the Advancement of Science (AAAS) in Chicago. Four of the contributors to this volume – Terry Bynum, Randy Miller, John Snapper, and I – made presentations. A special acknowledgment is owed to Elliot R. Siegel of the National Library of Medicine and the AAAS Section on Information, Computing, and Communication for encouraging this effort, and for his wise counsel.

The original idea for a book blossomed as it became increasingly clear that there was a major gap in the burgeoning literatures in bioethics and medical informatics. David A. Evans, a colleague in computational linguistics at Carnegie Mellon's Department of Linguistics and Philosophy, provided precious insight and vital encouragement. Richard Barling of Cambridge University Press recognized the opportunity to foster such a multidisciplinary effort, evincing saintly patience in the process.

Randy Miller, then of the University of Pittsburgh and now of Vanderbilt University, and a pioneer at the intersection of ethics, computing, and medicine, has been a mentor, a guide, and an advocate. Indeed, each of the contributors to this volume is owed a debt of gratitude. It is a rare opportunity to work with leading scholars with so diverse a set of backgrounds, and to be able to learn so much from them.

At the University of Miami, many people have provided a spectrum of support and made it possible, in one way or another, for this work to be completed. Special thanks are due Norman Altman, Lawrence Fishman, Diane Horner, John Masterson, and Steve Ullmann.

I am particularly indebted to my best teachers: Max, Jacqueline, Bob, Judith, and, especially, Allison.

K.W.G.
Forum for Bioethics and Philosophy
University of Miami, Miami

Contributors

Sheri A. Alpert, M.A., M.P.A.
Research Associate, The Institute of Public Policy
George Mason University
Fairfax, VA 22030

James G. Anderson, Ph.D.
Professor and Director, Social Research Institute
Department of Sociology and Anthropology
Purdue University
West Lafayette, IN 47907

Carolyn E. Aydin, Ph.D.
Assistant Administrtor for Nursing Research
Department of Nursing Practice, Research and Development
Cedars-Sinai Medical Center
8700 Beverly Blvd.
Los Angeles, CA 90048

Terrell Ward Bynum, Ph.D.
Director, Research Center on Computing and Society
Southern Connecticut State University
New Haven, CT 06515

John L. Fodor, Ph.D.
Research Associate, Research Center on Computing and Society
Southern Connecticut State University
New Haven, CT 06515

Kenneth W. Goodman, Ph.D.
Director, Forum for Bioethics and Philosophy
University of Miami
Miami, FL 33101

Randolph A. Miller, M.D.
Director, Biomedical Informatics
Vanderbilt University
Nashville, TN 37232

John W. Snapper, Ph.D.
Associate Dean of Science and Letters
Illinois Institute of Technology
Chicago, IL 60616

1

Bioethics and health informatics: an introduction

KENNETH W. GOODMAN

The intersection of bioethics and health informatics offers a rich array of issues and challenges for philosophers, physicians, nurses, and computer scientists. One of the first challenges is, indeed, to identify where the interesting and important issues lie, and how best, at least initially, we ought to address them. This introductory chapter surveys the current ferment in bioethics; identifies a set of areas of ethical importance in health informatics (ranging from standards, networks, and bioinformatics to telemedicine, epidemiology, and behavioral informatics); argues for increased attention to curricular development in ethics and informatics; and provides a guide to the rest of the book. Perhaps most importantly, this chapter sets the following tone: that in the face of extraordinary technological changes in health care, it is essential to maintain a balance between "slavish boosterism and hyperbolic skepticism." This means, in part, that at the seam of three professions we may find virtue both by staying up-to-date and by not overstepping our bounds. This stance is called "progressive caution." The air of oxymoron is, as ever in the sciences, best dispelled by more science.

A conceptual intersection

The future of the health professions is computational.

This suggests nothing quite so ominous as artificial doctors and robonurses playing out "what have we wrought?" scenarios in future cyberhospitals. It does suggest that the standard of care for information acquisition, storage, processing, and retrieval is changing rapidly, and health professionals need to move swiftly or be left behind. Because we are talking about health care, the stakes are quite high. The very idea of a standard of care in the context of pain, life, suffering, health, and death points directly to a vast ensemble of *ethical* issues. Failing to adhere to publicly defensible standards is to risk or do harm, which, without some overriding justification or reason, is unethical.

Indeed, medical informatics is rich with ethical issues. As we succeed

1

in hewing to a higher standard in health computing, we discover or come
to fear threats to privacy and confidentiality, risks of bias and discrimination, the danger of scientific and clinical hubris, the erosion of cherished
relationships, the degradation of precious skills. By responding to one
challenge, we create others. This is the case in the health sciences most
every time a new technology invites, compels, or seduces us: Dialysis,
organ transplantation, artificial organs, life support, genetic therapy, and
other advances all carry heavy social, financial, and ethical taxes. One
goal of this book is to add health informatics to the list of major technological innovations that simultaneously change practice and challenge
our values. Another goal is to begin to pay that moral tariff.

Ethical issues arise when we want to know what is right or wrong,
appropriate or inappropriate, praiseworthy or blameworthy, good or evil.
The study of right conduct and the practice of the healing professions are
ancient endeavors. It is a source of intellectual, social, and moral excite-
ment, then, that a wide-ranging ethical inquiry can be undertaken in the
domain of one of the most modern of human activities: the use of intelligent machines in the healing professions.

This book explores the intersection of three vast areas of inquiry: ethics,
computing, and medicine.[1] While each domain is huge, it is not yet clear
how large the intersection is. One might picture a Venn diagram with the
circles labeled "ethics," "medicine," and "computing." We already
have the two-way intersections or classes *medical ethics* (or more broadly
and accurately *bioethics*), *medical computing*, and *computing ethics*. This
volume is about the area formed by the bowed triangle at the center of
the diagram. Of course, it is not really the size of the intersection that we
care about, but its importance. It is a central supposition of this book that
the intersection is very important indeed. Throughout this chapter and the
book, the reader is presumed to be neither expert nor completely ignorant
of any of these fields. It would be a great misfortune if one had to be a
physician, computer scientist, *and* moral philosopher to draw from or contribute to our busy intersection.

This chapter has the task of providing an overview of this area of applied ethics, and setting the stage for the other contributions. The following

[1] Use of the terms "medicine" and "medical informatics" is intended to range across the
health professions. It is intended to include nursing and the behavioral sciences, for instance, which enjoy rapid development in, and have contributed extensively to, informatics.
It is a term of convenience and its use in this way is warranted by the tradition of including
nonmedical professions within its scope. It is used interchangeably with the term "health
informatics," though not "bioinformatics," which has come to be used in the context of
biotechnology and related disciplines.

sections in this chapter will address the current and tumultuous setting in bioethics; itemize and comment on a selection of the most salient issues at the intersection of ethics, computing, and medicine; offer a defense of ethics-and-informatics as an interdisciplinary domain worthy of educational emphasis and further research; and provide a conceptual map by which to locate the other chapters in the constellation of the several ethical issues.

What can bioethics do for health informatics?

The past quarter century has seen extraordinary growth in the field of bioethics. Philosophers, physicians, nurses, lawyers, epidemiologists, clergy, social workers, psychologists, health economists, policy makers, hospital administrators, and others have contributed to this growth. Some of the growth has been driven by the new medical technologies. The origin of the modern hospital ethics committee is often traced to the unhappily named ''God committees'' that apportioned access to dialysis machines in the 1960s. Today, genetics, organ procurement and allocation, and sophisticated life support techniques must be among the areas of competence for anyone who would practice clinical bioethics. Indeed, it is striking that there are people who identify themselves as ''bioethicists,'' and who are turned to as such in increasingly common reports in the popular media. The professional literature has accreted dramatically, with perhaps a dozen journals, extensive collections by major publishers, and several major professional societies.

Many nonphilosophers are interested in bioethics and related fields. One risks no hyperbole by saying that, in absolute and relative terms, more people are using a philosophical nomenclature (i.e., that of bioethics) than at any other time in the history of civilization. To be sure, there is a common tendency to do ethics by raising sequences of questions but failing to answer them; professional journals often feature papers on ethical topics which do little more than enumerate issues or questions. To write, ''Lo, an ethical issue'' is doubtless to make a contribution, often an important one. But it is insufficient.

There is also seemingly widespread ignorance among nonphilosophers about significant debates and disagreements over ethical theory, core concepts, and meta-ethics. These debates and their outcomes have major implications for professional practice.

In the two decades since the first edition of Tom L. Beauchamp and James F. Childress's *Principles of Biomedical Ethics,* the book has emerged as a conceptual and practical touchstone for a vast number of health professionals around the world. The volume is the closest thing bioethics has to a best seller, and its approach – the four-principles approach – comprises what are arguably the most widely recognized set of philosophical concepts ever: respect for autonomy, nonmaleficence, beneficence, and justice. One need not look far in the medical, nursing, psychological, epidemiological, health administration, or social work literatures to find these principles proffered as received knowledge in a settled domain, as in "There are four principles, and they are these. . . ."

This kind of approach is inadequate, ignorant of important other methods, and does a disservice to Beauchamp and Childress, who in the latest edition of their book provide an important response to proponents of alternative approaches (Beauchamp and Childress 1994). Several of those alternatives are important to identify here to give a flavor of the debate that is changing the shape of bioethics.

One key challenge to the four-principles approach has been crafted by the philosopher Bernard Gert. His system of morality identifies and develops a set of moral rules and moral ideals. The rules "form the core of a public system that applies to all rational persons," where rationality is in part the promotion of good and the avoidance of evil (Gert 1989; see Clouser and Gert 1990 for a critique of the four-principles approach and to appreciate the scope and seriousness of the debate). Gert's system is robust and captures a number of important intuitions about right and wrong.

Casuistry, or case-based analogical reasoning (Jonsen and Toulmin 1988), commands attention because of its accessibility in a wide variety of professional contexts and because many people find it productive and gratifying to be able to reason from clear cases, in which rightness or wrongness is not in doubt, to more challenging and ambiguous cases.

Virtue ethics takes virtues and not duties or good consequences to be of fundamental moral importance. It customarily traces its origins to Aristotle. It has enjoyed a resurgence in recent years because in part of the work of several highly respected thinkers (e.g., Pellegrino and Thomasma 1993).

Rights-based theories, which emphasize various kinds of human rights (Rawls 1971; Dworkin 1977), attempt to identify the moral and social sources of valid claims or entitlements, and, often, corresponding duties.

Communitarianism (MacIntyre 1981; Callahan 1994) takes communal or collective values to be the fount of rightness, and emphasizes the importance of shared social goals, of convention, and of tradition.

Additionally, there is much interest in feminist ethics (Holmes and Purdy 1992), and "care ethics" in nursing (Benjamin and Curtis 1992; Loewy 1995), where traditional rationality is demoted alongside human relationships and emotions, which are regarded as superior approaches to ethical and clinical problems.

These are, we may summarize, fertile time for bioethics. Most of the approaches itemized here have been applied to (or tried against) leading issues in contemporary bioethics. Expanding debate accompanies the question of which approach is best or even how much the various approaches differ from each other in important ways on issues we care most about. This is a happy lesson for a project that seeks to add medical informatics to the plate of issues in bioethics: Never before have so many people been studying and teaching bioethics and related fields. Rich theoretical disputes, along with numerous efforts to sort out practical problems in daily decision making, produce an environment conducive to this kind of topical expansion.

The same is true in the other direction. If bioethics can accommodate informatics, then informatics must include bioethics. There is already evidence of such a willingness, and we will return to this matter later.

To answer our question, "What can bioethics do for health informatics?" we can offer the following: Bioethics provides an interdisciplinary framework and rich theoretical options. Its theoretical plurality notwithstanding, bioethics has succeeded remarkably well in a short time in identifying issues and finding or inventing optimal solutions to practical problems. And bioethics has a solid track record of curricular development in nursing and medical schools and in colleges of arts and sciences. That said, we must not move too quickly past the fact that the plurality in bioethics leaves us without an unambiguous or uncontroversial approach that might be adopted for our purpose.

Bioethics and medical informatics are the same age, more or less. Both are vigorous and attractive to diverse students. It is time to identify or create conceptual and intellectual anastomoses between these two areas of practice and inquiry. This book is the first major attempt to further that effort.

Areas of ethical importance in medical informatics

Everyone knows that electronic patient records pose difficult challenges to confidentiality. But other interesting and fundamentally important ethical issues arise in medical informatics. Subsequent chapters in this book identify and explore these core issues. It will be helpful first, though, to identify the areas or domains or (sub)fields in which these issues arise. For instance, confidentiality and its cousin, privacy, turn up in many places beside hospital-based electronic patient records: There are serious concerns about confidentiality protections in hospital, interhospital, and corporate networks; in telemedicine applications; and in genetic databases distinct from patient records.

The rest of this section provides a provisional typology of medical and nursing computing applications and domains in which ethical issues arise. It is too optimistic to hope that it should be exhaustive; too many variables change with rapidity in health informatics. Also, some issues recur between and among several domains; for instance, telemedicine would often be impossible without some sort of network, and yet it is here assigned its own section because it suggests distinctive ethical issues. Also, similar ethical issues sometimes recur in different domains, as when concerns about group stigma arise in genetics as well as epidemiology. Such connections represent the richness of the intersection of ethics, computing, and medicine. The following applications and domains are assigned their own chapters and so are not included here: decision-support systems (Chapter 6), outcomes tracking and prognostic scoring systems (Chapter 7), and meta-analysis (Chapter 8). Chapters 2 through 5 explore the broader issues of human values, accountability, evaluation, and confidentiality. Connections will be identified between this section's applications and domains on the one hand, and subsequent chapters' issues and themes on the other.

Errors, standards, and *"progressive caution"*

There are vastly many ways to err in the practice of medicine, law, nursing, engineering, psychology, etc. Not all errors are created equal, however. Malpractice is often determined by appeal to various *standards*; if, for instance, most physicians in a given locale perform a particular procedure a certain way, then one who has a bad outcome after performing it a different way is liable for having stepped thus out of line. If the physician attempts the procedure in the standard way but botches it, he or she is still liable for having strayed from the standard for success. What constitutes a standard is an interesting problem, and solving it has interesting consequences.

Suppose the use of medical computers evolves to the point that half of all practitioners employ them to good effect. Are those who do *not* use computers then providing substandard care? A version of this question was raised in 1985 by a physician, philosopher, and lawyer in an article that should be seen as the first significant attempt to link ethics, computing, and medicine (Miller, Schaffner, and Meisel 1985; for an earlier approach, see Szolovits and Pauker 1979; for another early and interesting contribution, see de Dombal 1987). It will not be obvious when we cross such a Rubicon. Some medical liability insurers now offer modest premium discounts for physicians who adopt certain computer systems for clinical records, drug interactions, and patient education (Borzo 1995), and it has been suggested that computer use in medical offices is good for risk management (Bartlett 1994). Other computerized tools are said to reduce unacceptable levels of human errors (Boon and Kok 1993; Mango 1994). Is all this to be understood as evidence of a shift in the standard of care? The question is important for our purposes because there are important ethical reasons why one should want to provide at least a minimum standard of care. These include obligations to minimize morbidity and mortality to the best of one's ability, where clinicians are presumed able to learn traditional and new techniques. We can put this very simply: There is an ethical obligation to provide a standard level of care because one thereby maximizes good outcomes for patients, or at least asymptotically approaches such maximal good. If a leech or cyclotron or aspirin or computer helps achieve this, so much the better, usually.

We can agree to this: The vast amounts of information that clinicians need to master, or at least process, render the unaided human inadequate to increasingly many of the tasks that shape professional practice (Sadegh-Zadeh 1989).

When technologies are inchoate, we probably do best to set the standard bar low. This is because we tend to lack conceptual confidence that the standard is truly standard-worthy. (One of the things wrong with outcomes research is that it too often engenders overhasty values for purported standards; see Chapter 7.) Where the bar is set is not generally an ethical question unless it can be shown that the standard-setting metric was corrupted for other purposes: placing the bar too low to avoid hard work, for instance; or too high, to limit competition. One good place to set the bar initially is at "safety," although even there there is room for variation (Fox 1993; Davies 1996).

For years, nurses have been aware of many of these issues, especially including professional attitudes and appropriate roles, and impact on practice (Adams 1986; Smoyak 1986; Barhyte 1987; Woolery 1990). The very idea of professionalism in medical informatics has itself attained maturity as the discipline has evolved (Heathfield and Wyatt 1995).

Society has an interest in health care standards. Faced with expanding use of decision-support systems, society might opt to regard these programs as devices that should be regulated, or made by law to adhere to a certain standard. Whether and how decision-support systems should be officially recognized as medical devices, which are customarily regulated by governments, has been a topic of debate for some time. In the United States, the Food and Drug Administration has begun receiving applications for market approval of devices that aid human decision making (Gamerman 1992; Hamilton 1995; Food and Drug Administration 1996).

Questions of standards arise in the context of networks and their maintenance and security, as well as in considering the education of people who would use any of a variety of informatics tools, and even in the evaluation process which provides data for standards in the first place. It is important to emphasize the role of *technical standards* in contributing to standards of care. Whether a communication standard is proprietary or "open" is the source of great controversy in industry (Betts 1990). Also, various forces in industry, academia, and elsewhere support the development and adoption of technical standards for knowledge representation (Ludemann 1994), decision support (Mercier 1990), data exchange (LaPorte 1994; Hammond 1995), and other functions. The evolution of international health networks in general (Glowniak and Bushway 1994), and establishment of the "Global Health Network," an alliance of health and telecommunication professionals (Laporte et al. 1994; Aaron et al. 1996), exemplify vast opportunities and present great challenges. Well-wrought standards minimize errors; therefore, users, manufacturers, governments, and others have an ethical obligation to develop such standards. Of course, identifying an ethical obligation is different, though not necessarily easier, than developing technical standards, even in computing.

Errors, particularly medical errors, raise fascinating questions about inductive inference, rule-following, public policy, and on and on. What counts as an error, what kinds of errors are possible, and methods for error detection and avoidance are the source of important research and reflection (Gorovitz and MacIntyre 1976; Bosk 1979; Paget 1988; Bogner 1994; Leape 1994). One of the greatest fears elicited by the rise of computational medicine and nursing is that use, or inappropriate use, of these computational tools will cause patients to come to grief. A thread that runs throughout this volume (especially see Chapters 3 and 8) is that the most appropriate course to take is one we may call "progressive caution": Medical informatics is, happily, here to stay, but users and society have extensive responsibilities to ensure that we use our tools appropriately. This might cause us to move more deliberately or slowly than some would like. Ethically speaking, that is just too bad.

Health information networks

Depending on one's goals, two computers are better than one. A thousand might be better still.

The last decade has seen the extraordinary proliferation of electronic links within, between, and among hospitals, health maintenance organizations, multispecialty groups, insurance companies, clinics, physicians' and nurses' offices, laboratories, research sites, pharmacies, and, indeed, any place that people visit for health care or related services and any place that stores information about those visits. Many such entities are represented on the Internet and the World Wide Web. It is not often clear where one network ends and another begins; there is even a sense in which it does not make sense to ask where one network ends or begins. Networks link places downtown and places in the boondocks. Electronic mail, including messages containing confidential patient information, are transmitted across offices and around the world on networks. (To appreciate the scope of and need for health data networks, see Parsons, Fleischer, and Greenes 1992. For a general account of issues for networked communities, see Denning and Lin 1994. For examples of community health information networks [CHINs], see Pemble 1994, and McGowan, Evans, and Michl 1995.)

The growth of national and international networks offers unprecedented opportunities, even as it suggests responsibilities not yet clearly understood. Canada's Health Net and the United States's Health Information Network (a National Information Infrastructure project) are examples of attempts to connect disparate entities in the service of public health.

More modestly, consider Patient X, a 35-year-old homosexual man. He goes to his physician for a physical exam and, during the interview, allows as how he fears he might have contracted the human immunodeficiency virus. The physician records this information on a hand-held device that transmits it to the group-practice computer, along with the patient's weight, blood pressure, the fact that he had a tonsillectomy 30 years ago, and so on. (The device prompted the physician when he forgot which questions to ask.) He orders an HIV test. Now what constitutes appropriate use of this information? Note that there are yet no results of the test – all that is on the record is the fact that a test has been ordered. The physician might use this information to counsel X about safe sex, and the insurance company might use it to reimburse the physician for conducting the exam. But the physician might also share the information with a pharmacy that wants to market a new anti-retroviral drug, or a university that is seeking data for a behavioral medicine study. Or, the insurance company might decide to drop X from its plan because the need for the test itself suggests the patient has risk factors which increase the chance he will one day require expensive treatment. Such concerns, most common in the United States, are arising with increasing frequency in Europe (Whitney 1996). Do the developers, owners, maintainers, or users of the *network* confront ethical issues here, or just those who make decisions about referrals, or research, or current or future reimbursement?

There might be no question at all about confidentiality – suppose X authorized review of his records by third-party payers (as do most people hoping their treatment will be paid for). Or there might be such questions if, for instance, X did not know of the possible consequences of his authorization.

Let us propose several ways to view the moral status of health information networks:

- *Networks are value neutral.* Here, networks are mere media, like television or radio, such that it does not make any sense to say that they are good or bad in themselves. On this model, networks themselves raise no ethical issues. Ethical scrutiny is appropriate only in evaluating the uses to which their information is put.
- *Networks are value laden.* One might liken networks (for the sake of example) to weapons and suggest that, once we are aware of the possible uses of the things, we must examine the intentions of those who designed and built them. In this case, a network developer cannot dust off his or her hands and declaim that an evil entity (insurance company, HMO, government, university, etc.) is to blame for any ensuing wrongdoing.
- *Networks are shared-value entities.* This is an "all of the above" model, configured to assign moral responsibility to all who build *and* use a network. Developers who failed to create and evaluate access, authentication, and other security measures cannot adopt a self-righteous stance and blame hackers who compromise a network for evil purposes. Neither, however, can the hackers shirk responsibility for evildoing. If pa-

tient X loses his insurance, we can go so far as to fault society for failing to establish adequate safeguards. (This assumes we regard it as wrong that sick people be denied health coverage because they are sick, a concern all the more pressing given the current inclination to blame people for their illnesses.) This model seems quite attractive, but key points would require additional development.

Networks and various storage media also provide the data that fuel much institutional, scientific, economic, and policy-driven outcomes research. If a managed care organization uses networked databases to calculate outcomes, thus to guide decision making about whether clinical referrals will be endorsed, it is clear that we need to weigh the following carefully: benefits to society from reduced referrals to expensive specialists; erosion of the autonomy and decision-making authority of the referring physician or nurse; and risks of undertreatment when making an inference from (1) a general guideline or rule to (2) the best treatment plan in a particular case.

The issues we have identified under this heading include these: What values are central and which peripheral in designing, building, and using health information systems? How is responsibility for harms best established? When has there been enough evaluation? These questions are precisely those taken up in the subsequent three chapters and Chapter 8.

Do-it-yourself health care

Publicly accessible health networks and off-the-shelf decision-support systems may be viewed as occupying a spectrum that ranges between the following two extremes: (1) A great and democratizing service that decentralizes health care and empowers patients, or (2) a silly and dangerous way to allow people to practice medicine and nursing without licenses. If we intermix the increasing availability of on-line consultations we can envision cyberspace as including a health care neighborhood right next to, or even as part of, entertainment and commerce.

On-line patient self-help resources and decision aids are quite popular. In the United States, the National Cancer Institute maintains sites that attract 200,000 users a month, and one on-line service reports that 6 percent of users said a health site helped them avoid an emergency department visit and 26 percent said it helped them avoid a physician's visit (Gilbert 1996). Some 30,000 people started taking an epilepsy drug for amyotrophic lateral sclerosis, a disease for which it was not approved, because it was touted in on-line discussion groups (Bulkeley 1995). Hundreds of thousands of people have visited DeathNET, a Canadian web site on death and dying, including suicide (Lessenberry 1996).

On-line patient instruction and information materials are distributed by health care providers to patients or accessed directly by patients from the Internet (Ferguson 1995). The prospect of comprehensive, easily accessible, up-to-date, and salient patient information is glorious . . . as long as it does not substitute for or interfere with therapeutically efficacious provider-patient relationships, does not contribute to dangerous misunderstandings, and does not elicit a mistaken sense of security. (On the question of computer-mediated changes in the professional-patient relationship, see Kluge 1993.) What computers promise in speed, ease, and scope, humans must guarantee by quality control and hard work. Journeys through the World Wide Web are often noteworthy for the number of unfinished, abandoned, and outdated sites. We should insist on more than clinical hope, or intentions, to guarantee the quality of these materials. Patient materials might best be considered a form of journalism: Well-earned reputations for quality will earn the greatest number of subscribers. Put this way, it is clear that quality control and error avoidance are the leading ethical issues that arise here.

One mechanism for addressing these issues is peer review. But it is not clear how much peer review is necessary or even how to evaluate such review. One well-known, on-line oncology information resource, OncoLink (Buhle, Goldwein, and Benjamin 1994), was the locus of an extensive dispute over the quality of material. The University of Pennsylvania took control of the service away from a Ph.D. scientist who founded it and gave control to co-founding M.D.s, apparently in part because the former had made available the text of newspaper articles that had not been peer reviewed. One of the points of this dispute turns on the question of who is an appropriate peer.

A similar problem arises with on-line support groups (Lamberg 1996). A seemingly innocuous outlet for people with shared miseries might dissuade patients who need professional treatment. The problem is not that free people are taking control of their own health care; it is that ignorant people or people misled by unrealistic hope will mistake comfort or gossip for skilled medical, nursing, or psychological help.

But what about on-line consultations by appropriate professionals? In one notable case, a woman in China was comatose after a variety of central nervous system symptoms. After tests ruled out a number of diagnoses and she failed to respond well to treatment, Beijing University students sent e-mail around the world asking for diagnostic help. All told, there were more than 2,000 responses, with one of the early ones rendering the correct diagnosis, thallium poisoning (Gunby 1995).

Rendering diagnoses without being able to touch, hear, or see the person being diagnosed? Well, we should say that the proof will be in the pudding. If professionals are able to make remote diagnoses and provide electronic advice with at least the accuracy and quality of more traditional means, then we should be morally delighted at this good turn of events. Leaving aside the problem of how one would ethically test such a system, it remains unclear how one ventures to render such a diagnosis in the first place. If one is trying to help confounded physicians in Beijing or Birmingham or Boston, or if there is some sort of emergency, or in the absence of other, more customary alternatives – well, that is one thing. But to provide advice and diagnoses by e-mail is to risk error with questionable justification. We require reasons, or, better, *good* reasons, to deviate from an independently evolved standard of care. Without such warrant, we risk recklessness, or worse.

Telemedicine, telesurgery, and virtual reality

In less than a decade, telemedicine has grown into an extraordinary international enterprise, with scientists, clinicians, governments, and entrepreneurs striving to create remote-presence health care (Preston 1994; De Maeseneer and Beolchi 1995; Ferguson, Doarn, and Scott 1995; Lipson 1995). One early and widely quoted consulting report suggested that telemedicine could be used to provide health care to millions of people and save hundreds of millions of dollars (Arthur D. Little, Inc. 1992). Telemedicine, or the use of a variety of video, audio, and other tools to examine distant patients, or images of them, is seen as a way to provide health care to those otherwise unblessed: people in rural areas, on battlefields, in space. It also provides a means for experts in one place to help colleagues in another, as when a family practitioner in the country wants a radiologist in the city to help interpret an X-ray (Franken et al. 1992). Radiology, dermatology, and pathology – the most visual of the medical sciences – are already employing telemedical tools on a regular basis. Dermatologists, for instance, often examine prisoners in other buildings or cities, and tests have included specialists in orthopedics, urology, pediatrics, ophthalmology, and physical therapy (e.g., Delaplain, Lindborg, Norton, and Hastings 1993).

In surgery, there has been great progress in computer-assisted surgical planning, dexterity enhancement, surgical robots and autopilots, and "telepresence surgery," or the use of remote control surgical tools (Taylor et al. 1996).

There have been the first stirrings of interest in the ethical issues that arise in telemedicine (Norton, Lindborg, and Delaplain 1993; Allaërt and Dusserre 1995; Goodman 1996a), but technical and business aspects have outstripped them. What are the ethical issues here? Obviously, we need to learn more about how telemedicine compares to traditional approaches; in the absence of data showing that patients are at least as well off after telemedical encounters (or compelling reasons to demote these concerns, as in emergencies), we must attach the highest importance to error avoidance and the question of an emerging standard of care. Such data are being collected in many arenas, as for instance in interpretation of digitized images in dermatopathology (Perednia, Gaines, and Butruille 1995), and are encouraging. But as elsewhere in the history of medicine, a new tool is slowly being adopted at the same time as it is being tested and evaluated. By the time we have amassed sufficient data to warrant extensive use of new tools, the use has already become a *fait accompli.*

Concerns about confidentiality and valid consent are paramount, as is the following: While we should be delighted that prisoners or people in rural areas will receive health care, we need to ensure that we do not use telemedicine to let us off the hook too easily. If there is a difficulty in enticing physicians and nurses to practice in rural areas, then it is not clear that we should pretend to overcome this difficulty by providing telemedicine services. Clinicians might just have a moral obligation to practice where they are needed. This is an especially important point until such time as telemedicine has been adequately evaluated and a minimal standard of care rigorously described.

It should be remarked that this book is nearly bereft of predictions about the future of computing and telecommunications. Such predictions constitute a tempting but nugatory hobby, one which is usually as hollow as it is popular. One exception will be permitted here: The explosion in home care, which, like many changes in health care nowadays is undertaken primarily in hopes it will conserve resources while maintaining quality, will be made ever more cost effective if home care physicians and nurses do not need to go to their patients' homes. Telemedicine will accelerate this trend. Rapid advances in picture-phone technology, for instance, will make home care as easy as telephoning a patient. Ease and quality of practice are distinct, of course, and should be evaluated distinctly.

The development of virtual reality in medicine is another exciting phenomenon, although, as with many other exciting modern phenomena, most of the goods are contained in promissory notes (cf. Kaltenborn and Rien-hoff 1993). As with many new technologies, it is not always clear how even to define core terms or identify their scope. It will be sufficient to define virtual reality as the use of computers to fashion sensory or cognitive analogs to actual experiences. Applied in the health professions, it allows one in principle to "view" or "touch" a lifelike simulacrum of a person or animal. This has its clearest use in educational settings (Merril 1994). Appropriately outfitted with sensory headset and gloves, a surgery student can perform a virtual cardiac catheterization or laparoscopy, or examine, prepare, and operate on a virtual patient. He or she would see the virtual patient's abdomen, feel the proxy scalpel pass through apparent skin and fascia, and discover that an illusory appendix had ruptured or a cancer metastasized. A virtual tumor could then be resected, with feedback loops creating the impression that real tissue appeared a certain way, that it was oriented in such-and-such a way to surrounding tissue and organs, and that, when cut, it could be removed. If the student erred and nicked an artery or bowel, there would be an opportunity to do an emergency repair. If the patient happened to die, this unhappy turn of events would contribute to the learning experience. (The student might then use the Psychiatry Department's communication expert system to tell the virtual family that virtual grandmother had bitten the virtual dust.) Educational prospects for virtual reality in the health professions may be compared to the use of flight simulators in aviation. These have attained a high degree of sophistication and are used extensively to train pilots. But whether such tools can maintain or improve professional training levels remains an open question. Their use in practice pits risks and potential benefits against each other in a delicate tension (*Lancet* 1991).

It has also been suggested that virtual reality might be of direct use in psychiatric and psychological patient care. A patient would don a headset and enter a sensory parallel world which could be altered for therapeutic purposes. A phobic might, for instance, be made to confront seemingly veridical instantiations of the object of his fear and, in experiencing no physical harm, overcome the phobia (Lamson 1995). It has been suggested that virtual reality systems might be used for neuropsychology evaluations and neural prostheses to reduce sensory impairment – and subsequently perhaps to reduce reliance on medication, or even to modify behavior (Whalley 1995).

It is not clear how one might ethically conduct a rigorous trial to test the safety or efficacy of such uses. It is uncontroversially unethical to use or presume the value of such a gadget without such tests. In general, the correct stance to take when contemplating such proto-tools is to be on guard against slavish boosterism and hyperbolic skepticism, and to scrutinize existing research and development.

Bioinformatics

When scientists in Cambridge, England, and St. Louis, Missouri, wanted to make 900,000 nucleotide bases publicly available so colleagues around the world could join the effort to locate and identify a breast cancer gene, they did not publish a book, airmail parcels of human tissue, or pick up the telephone. They placed the sequence data on two publicly accessible file transfer protocol sites on the Internet (Dickson 1995). The gene sequences themselves are identified computationally. And the sequences are rendered tractable in comparative sequence analyses by the method of data base homology searching (Boguski 1995). In other words, genes are discovered, sequenced, shared, and analyzed with computers. On-line genetic databases have been likened to a new form of communication among scientists (Hilgartner 1995).

It could not be otherwise. There is far too much information to be managed by pre-computational media. The evolution of genetic databases and tools for searching them is proceeding so rapidly that scientists are building computational toolkits to hold their computational tools (Miller et al. 1995; Waldrop 1995; Williams 1995).

Too, geneticists have developed databases that include clinical information, photographic material, pedigree, and gene localization data. This information is analyzed by computer to "facilitate diagnosis and further gene localization" (Arena and Lubs 1991).

While the ethical issues that arise in genetic research, testing, and therapy are the source of much research and are increasingly well understood (Annas and Elias 1992; Andrews et al. 1994; Frankel and Teich 1994), the addition of informatics and information retrieval makes clear that we must attend to an expanded cluster of issues. These issues include data sharing, quality control, group and subgroup stigma, and privacy and confidentiality, including the idea of "group confidentiality" (Goodman 1996b). The inclusion of genetic information in electronic medical records opens a new frontier in bioethics, computing ethics, and health informatics. It scarcely needs mention that bioinformatics has taken the course it has in part because of the availability of extensive networks; hence, issues that apply in discussing the role of networks will often apply here as well.

The rise of bioethics as a professional and academic discipline has been of use, interest, and/or importance in a variety of other fields. When areas of research and practice are new, as is the case with telemedicine and bioinformatics, the contributions of bioethics can in principle be all the greater. That people practice bioinformatics or study or teach it is itself a reason to include an ethics component. The evidence from other domains is that practitioners need it, students enjoy it, and society derives nontrivial benefits from such efforts.

Epidemiology and public health

Let us introduce a term, "computational epidemiology," to refer to the use of computers to identify correlations between events, behaviors, predispositions, environments, and other physiological, social, and behavioral antecedent conditions on one hand, and disease, morbidity, and mortality on the other. Creation and analysis of public health data, especially in very large databases, is a computational task. Some public health databases contain clinical information and thus are rich sources of knowledge (Safran and Chute 1995). There are periodic calls for integrated, comprehensive health data surveillance and storing systems (LaPorte et al. 1994; Thacker and Stroup 1994). Information processing tools can also correct measurement errors, as for risk estimates (Bashir and Duffy 1995). And automated monitoring, as of pollution-mediated disease, holds the prospect of vast computational health surveillance networks (Brooks et al. 1993).

Ethical tensions in epidemiology are among the most philosophically interesting in all bioethics, and the subfield of ethics and epidemiology is enjoying a surge of important scholarly work (e.g., Coughlin and Beauchamp 1996). Epidemiology's philosophical challenges tend to come from the philosophy of science, and include induction, confirmation, and causation (see the discussions of outcomes in Chapter 7 and meta-analysis in Chapter 8). For our purposes, it will be sufficient to suggest that these issues constitute a rich source of cases of decision making in contexts marked by scientific uncertainty (see Szolovits 1995). Suppose a statistical analysis of data in a large, on-line cancer (or birth-defect) registry suggests a correlation between elevated cancer rates (or birth defects) and habitation near a waste processing plant. Should – and how should – scientists communicate these correlations to people who will want to know if the plant *causes* cancer or birth defects? Do residents need to understand the structure of the database, knowledge representation protocol, or statistical methods? What is the role of the popular media in communicating possible risks? These questions are answered by appeal to core values and by attending to the possibility and consequences of making an error that in one way or another involves the use of a computer. To be sure, these problems existed before computers. But compared to earlier methods, computational processing of electronic databases creates a difference in kind by virtue of a difference in magnitude.

Additionally, statistical analysis itself raises ethical issues: of data selection, management, and sharing; publication and authorship; and scientific interpretation and truth telling (Derr 1994). Here, however, it is not as clear that the introduction of a computer has raised new issues or magnified old ones (a notable exception being meta-analysis).

In addition to error avoidance, computational epidemiology elevates concerns about confidentiality and valid consent to new levels. If patient records linked to unique identifiers are the source of data, it is necessary to overcome a number of obstacles to obtaining consent and ensuring confidentiality. But even if the records are – or are rendered – unlinked, there are still difficult issues. The issue of "group confidentiality" and stigma arises anew and ranges across all human diseases (Gostin 1991; Coughlin 1996); genetic, ethnic, or racial information introduces challenges we have only just begun to analyze (Roberts 1992; Lock 1994). Such analysis is essential as molecular or genetic epidemiology progresses and adopts ever-more-sophisticated information processing tools.

Behavioral informatics

There is a rich history of computer use in psychology and psychiatry. ELIZA, the computer program that played psychiatrist and attempted to model psychotherapy interactions (Weizenbaum 1976), captured the imagination of a generation of clinicians and scientists, many of whom reckoned that the behavioral sciences lent themselves especially well to computational decision support, if not emulation. Today, computers are used for patient or client tracking, assessment and testing, therapy and counseling, decision support, and other purposes (Wilkins 1994). To the extent that research in artificial intelligence attempts to model or replicate human cognition or reasoning skills, there is a sense, albeit controversial, in which much work in computer science may be regarded as doing research in psychology.

Ethical issues in behavioral informatics parallel those in clinical medicine and nursing, although it is worth emphasizing that confidentiality issues need to be addressed with increased gravity owing to the especially sensitive nature of psychological or psychiatric records. Indeed, the mere fact that someone has sought psychological or psychiatric assistance is itself potentially stigmatizing.

Attention to ethical issues at the intersection of computing and mental health began more than a decade ago and has tended to emphasize confidentiality and privacy, professional standards, therapy, and most recently care management (Colby 1986; Wolkon and Lyon 1986; Adman and Foster 1988; Ford 1993; Brown and Kornmayer 1996). Mental health patients constitute a vulnerable population; such populations are customarily regarded as entitled to increased protections. Our concerns for error avoidance and care standards loom especially large here. Issues related to valid or informed consent are also of special concern for behavioral medicine patients: To what extent is it reasonable to expect that any patients, let alone those with cognitive deficits or emotional trauma, say, should be informed about the role of intelligent machines in their care and treatment? That the answer to this question is not known is taken in Chapter 6 to constitute support for the idea of progressive caution.

Other issues

This section is reserved so we may itemize some additional applications which command attention but which in whole or in part do not fall neatly under the other headings. (The use of computers and networks for ethics education itself [e.g., Sieghart and Dawson 1987; Goodman 1992; Derse and Krogull 1994] is outside the scope of our discussion.)

Advance directives in electronic medical records. A complete and accurate patient chart is among the cornerstones of standard clinical practice. Advance directives, including living wills, are used with increasing frequency by patients to make their wishes known in case they later become incompetent or unable to communicate; this is generally a salutary development. Inclusion of such documents in electronic records raises the question whether they improve respect for advance directives, in part by serving as a sort of ethical reminder protocol. Enough data exist to suggest they do (Dexter, Gramelspacher, Wolinsky, Zhou, and Tierney 1996), but this requires additional study. One concern might be that electronic advance directives support the awful phenomenon in which health professionals reduce caring and other support of patients who want to refuse only heroic measures but not other treatments or procedures.

Monitoring, interviewing, and data capture. Handheld devices with links to hospital mainframes, continuous critical care monitoring, off-site telemetry (including implant and device tracking), and other ways to gather and store information are changing the shape of clinical and hospital practice. They are included here because, in addition to the familiar issues of confidentiality, standard of care, and, perhaps, skill degradation, they should be evaluated in terms of their effects on the physician- or nurse-patient relationship. Any tool that erodes that relationship, as for instance by impeding or superseding direct human communication, is worrisome (Goodman 1993). This can be an issue even in contexts where patients are unconscious if the use of monitoring or automatic data-capture tools reduces efficacious expert human attention. Also, computers have been used to monitor patient compliance with health maintenance plans (Frame et al. 1994), which some patients might find intrusive.

Case management. Patient case management, perhaps especially for diabetics, offers a number of opportunities for computational assistance (Albisser 1989; Albisser, Meneghini, and Mintz 1996). Controlling diabetes can be an extraordinary clinical challenge, and computational and telematic approaches bid fair to improve outcomes. Ethical issues arise if there is confusion over the status of the computer in the management. If professionals are unclear about the use of computers in health care, then surely patients will be forgiven if they lose track of the fact that ''computational case management'' is a figure of speech and that professionals, not computers, actually manage cases.

Organ transplant registries and allocation. Computers have become essential for organ registries, or databases of organ donors, recipients, and potential recipients. Computers are used to make donor-recipient matches and rank recipients on the basis of need, compatibility, prognosis, etc. (Wikler 1989), and to record the wishes of potential donors and make this information quickly and widely available (Salaman, Griffin, Ross, and Haines 1994). While it is unlikely that computer registries either worsen or solve the ethical problems associated with allocation of this scarce resource, it is important to be on guard against the illusion of objectivity that computer use can project. If an allocation protocol is unfair, the computer cannot make it fair.

Machine translation and informed consent. Most physicians in Paris do not understand Arabic, most in London are ignorant of Urdu, and most in New York are incompetent in Spanish. Hospital interpreters (of spoken language) and translators (of texts) are in increasing demand as communities grow more diverse. The need for reliable, accurate inter-language communication is essential for clinical encounters and research. For instance, suppose a randomized trial in Miami plans to recruit Anglo, Hispanic, and Haitian patients. This research cannot proceed if the documents and process for valid consent do not make it easy for all subjects to understand the aims, risks, and alternatives to participation. We have made great progress in the use of computers to translate natural language, and it is not remarkable to turn to natural language processing (perhaps including voice recognition) to help in the informed consent process. Our ethical attention is drawn to the following issues: the erosion of the consent process, accuracy and standards, and impediments to clinical relationships (Goodman 1996c).

It is sometimes said in bioethics that all clinical cases, even the boring ones, have an ethical component. This is a useful educational heuristic, and it may be pressed without trivializing our concerns by spreading them too broadly, or thinly. We should advance the same point in medical informatics: All uses of computers in the health professions raise ethical issues. Some command greater attention than others, and many, perhaps, are straightforward and easy to address and resolve. Creative application of this view should serve us well as new ways are devised to use computers and related devices in the service of human health.

Education in ethics and informatics

Worldwide, there are now dozens of training programs in medical and nursing informatics. One may receive undergraduate and postgraduate training, including doctorates, in informatics. Additionally, the number of conferences, colloquia, symposia, and certificate programs is vast and available on most continents. Education and informatics are natural partners (Friedman and Dev 1996). Yet unlike other scientific and medical programs, informatics training rarely includes attention to ethical issues, or, if it does, it tends to emphasize confidentiality, privacy, and legal issues to the exclusion of other core issues.

This is no longer adequate.

There are a number of arguments for greater attention to ethics in informatics training. First, ethical issues are important and recognized as such in affiliated fields. One should no more omit ethics from a medical school curriculum than physiology or cell biology. The issues affect practice and are ubiquitous, and attention to them produces better-rounded practitioners.

Second, the issues are interesting. Ethical issues are among the greatest challenges for physicians, nurses, and psychologists. It is frequently the case that scientific challenges (how to intubate or resuscitate a patient) are easy compared to the ethical challenges (*whether* to intubate or resuscitate). The inclusion of social issues makes for an especially exciting addition to the curriculum.

Third, ethics education provides practical guidance. One goal of applied ethics is to improve decision making in the professions. If it is the case that ethical challenges are sometimes at least as difficult as scientific ones, then there must be a pedagogical mechanism to help produce ethically optimized decisions. The richness of ethical debate and argumentation serves to improve real-world decision making.

The growth and proliferation of informatics programs in colleges and universities provide many opportunities to include attention to ethical issues in the curriculum at the outset, or at least early on. At the University of Miami, for instance, a new curriculum in medical informatics and telemedicine includes a component in social and ethical issues. Even in individual hospitals there are opportunities to address ethical issues in informatics; institutional ethics committees are ideally situated to begin such efforts.

Professional societies can contribute. This volume grew out of a session on ethics and informatics at the 1992 meeting of the American Association for the Advancement of Science in Chicago. In 1994 in Miami Beach the Annual Session of the American College of Physicians included a workshop (in conjunction with the American Medical Informatics Association [AMIA]) titled "Ethics and Responsibility in Medical Computing: Guidelines for Practitioners." Also that year, in Washington, AMIA's Fall Symposium featured a panel discussion on "Ethics and Informatics"; and the First World Congress on Computational Medicine, Public Health, and Biotechnology, meeting in Austin, Texas, included a session with several presentations on ethical issues. In 1996 in Washington, AMIA sponsored a Fall Symposium tutorial on "Ethical and Social Challenges for Medical Informatics."

It is always a challenge to include new components in established curricula. Yet informatics can look to other fields for models. In epidemiology, for instance, attention to ethical issues has increased dramatically in a comparatively short time (as curricular changes go), and courses in ethics and epidemiology are available at a number of universities and employ a variety of curricular materials (Goodman and Prineas 1996). Further, existing programs might easily be modified to include ethical issues. Institutions that offer programs or short courses in research integrity or the responsible conduct of science can be arranged to include components in bioinformatics and meta-analysis, for instance.

In the other direction: The bioethics curriculum has matured to the point that in addition to core issues such as end-of-life issues, confidentiality, organ transplantation, valid consent, resource allocation, and so on, it also includes somewhat more esoteric issues, ranging from xenographic transplantation to the handling of frozen embryos. Surely ethical issues raised by health care's omnipresent new computational tools merit inclusion in the bioethics canon. Some of the issues, such as confidentiality, will be familiar ones with new twists; others, such as appropriate use of decision-support systems, can provide exciting and novel challenges to core values and theoretical or meta-ethical stances.

It is time to develop a model curriculum for ethics and informatics. This could include both text-based and multimedia learning opportunities. Interactive experiences would be a natural adjunct to an ethics and informatics course. A diverse faculty could be drawn from computing, medicine, nursing, philosophy, psychology, and elsewhere. Such a curriculum could, in its instantiation in the burgeoning number of informatics programs, capture a lesson learned repeatedly in a broad range of professional training courses and schools:

Long after their training is completed, students tend to remember and be influenced by values far more than by facts.

Guide to the book

Our goal in this chapter has been to provide an overview of the intersection of ethics, medicine, and computing. We began by looking at the intersections of bioethics and medical informatics and discovered two disciplines in ferment. We concluded that the former had much to offer the latter. We then reviewed a number of areas of ethical importance in informatics: networks; errors and standards; ''do-it-yourself health care''; telemedicine, telesurgery, and virtual reality; bioinformatics; epidemiology and public health; behavioral informatics; and miscellaneous issues. In what follows, this discussion will be developed in terms of central concepts (Chapters 2, 3, 4, and 5) and special applications (Chapters 6, 7, and 8).

In Chapter 2, Terry Bynum, a founder of the field of computer ethics, and his colleague at Southern Connecticut State University, Jerry Fodor, provide a broad conceptual setting in which to view use of computers in medicine. By attending to human goals writ large, they locate informatics in the context of core values. One of their approaches, derived from the seminal work of Jim Moor (Moor 1979) at Dartmouth College, is to ask the fundamental question, "Are there health-related tasks we must not let computers perform?" Their answer serves as a valuable guide for an exciting new science.

John Snapper of the Illinois Institute of Technology, and another founder of computer ethics, extends his work on responsibility in computing by offering in Chapter 3 an analysis of accountability and moral liability, and suggesting a distinctive and robust approach to health computing responsibility for humans and their machines.

Chapter 4, by James G. Anderson of Purdue and Carolyn Aydin of Cedars-Sinai Medical Center in Los Angeles, makes the crucial point that system evaluation is a necessary component of successful implementation and, as such, constitutes an *ethical* imperative. Anderson and Aydin, who for years have been at the vanguard of research on health computer system evaluation, argue that systems must be evaluated in their context of use, and that failure to do so is ethically blameworthy.

In Chapter 5, Sheri Alpert of George Mason University gives a comprehensive survey of issues and problems related to confidentiality and argues that policy makers and system designers and users must attach as much importance to privacy and confidentiality as they do to patient outcomes, treatment records, or prescription tracking.

Chapter 6 reviews ethical issues associated with the use of decision-support systems. Randolph Miller of Vanderbilt University, a pioneer in both medical informatics and work on associated ethical issues, and I hold that a traditional understanding of appropriate tool use in health care confers a strong and practical obligation on system users.

Use of computers in outcomes research, especially in severity scoring systems, is analyzed in Chapter 7. I argue that outcome and prognostic scoring systems are recent phenomena and that inferences about quality of care and clinical prognoses must be weighed against the fact of the techniques' youth and attendant controversy; and in any case that they are not valid substitutes for clinico-ethical decision making and fair health care policy making. Clinicians and policy makers must take special precautions to prevent inappropriate use of outcomes studies and practice guidelines in the care of individual patients.

Chapter 8 suggests that the use of computational meta-analysis raises fundamental ethical issues related to the clinical applications of scientific research. It is concluded that, like many computational tools in the health professions, meta-analysis should be applied only with extreme caution and a thoroughgoing understanding of how the tool works.

Conclusion

As year succeeds year, some new physical or chemical technic and some new and elaborate machine are applied to the study of disease; great claims are always made for the precision of the answers yielded by these technics and machines. One of the greatest struggles that a practicing doctor has is to keep up-to-date with advances of this kind. No sooner has he mastered one than another is upon him. Moreover, the machines or technics are often so complex that he cannot understand them. He has to take what they tell him on trust. It must be within the experience of many of us that there is a growing tendency for doctors to rely on the information given by such technics and machines in preference to the information which they gain themselves from the history and physical signs. I am extremely doubtful that this is in the interests of good doctoring, and for three reasons. First, the errors and limitations of these new technics are not at first appreciated. Often the data yielded by clinical examination are of much greater precision in the identification of disease. Second, a thorough clinical examination, which will be carried out only by doctors who appreciate its worth, is the best method of establishing that spirit of mutual understanding and good will which is the core of the doctor-patient relationship. Finally, to rely on data, the nature of which one does not understand, is the first step in losing intellectual honesty. The doctor is peculiarly vulnerable to a loss of this kind, since so much of therapeutics is based on suggestion. And the loss naturally leaves him and his patients poorer (Pickering 1955).

These remarks by George W. Pickering, M.D., of London, come from his Convocation Address to the 36th Annual Session of American College of Physicians in Philadelphia more than 40 years ago. They are instructive on a number of counts, not least because they capture the stance taken throughout this book. Good doctoring and nursing are *human* skills; while those skills increasingly require augmentation of the sort offered by information storage and processing systems, the systems have no such skills.

Consider a traffic accident. A helicopter arrives with emergency medical technicians who administer first aid and attach monitoring devices to the injured driver. While the helicopter is returning to the hospital, telemetry systems are feeding the monitoring data to a computer in the hospital. Witness accounts and information about the kind of automobile, angle of incidence, use of seatbelts, and so forth are also transmitted to the hospital, where staffers at a physician's workstation identify a number of possible internal injuries. A decision-support system calculates the relative likelihood of each of several differential diagnoses, and alerts appropriate surgical specialists. By the time the patient arrives at the trauma center a severity scoring system has estimated the his chances of survival. Of course, his electronic medical record immortalizes him as a datum to be used in estimating the chance of success of treating others just like him.

What is sometimes called "ubiquitous medical computing" is the evolution of a computational cocoon that surrounds increasingly many patients in increasingly many situations. A goal of this book is to address our obligations and our entitlements in a world in which an ancient science meets the most modern and perhaps the most powerful of man's creations.

References

Aaron, D.J., Sekikawa, A., Libman, I.M., Iochida, L., Barinas-Mitchell, E., and LaPorte, R.E. 1996. Telepreventive medicine. *M.D. Computing* 13: 335–8.

Adams, G.A. 1986. Computer technology: its impact on nursing practice. *Nursing Administration Quarterly* 10(2): 21–33.

Adman, H.P., and Foster, S.W. 1988. Ethical issues in the use of computer-based assessment. *Computers in Human Services* 3: 71–87.

Albisser, A.M. 1989. Intelligent instrumentation in diabetic management. *CRC Critical Reviews in Biomedical Engineering* 17: 1–24.

Albisser, A.M., Meneghini, L.M., and Mintz, D.H. 1996. New on-line computer system for daily diabetes intervention: first year experience (abstract). *Diabetes* 46 (Suppl. 2): 71A.

Allaërt, F.-A., and Dusserre, L. 1995. Télémédecine et responsabilité médicale. *Archives d Anatomie et de Cytologie Pathologiques* 43: 200–5.

Andrews, L.B., Fullarton, J.E., Holtzman, N.A., and Motulsky, A.G. eds. 1994. *Assessing Genetic Risks: Implications for Health and Social Policy.* Washington, D.C: National Academy Press.

Annas, G.J., and Elias, S. eds. 1992. *Gene Mapping: Using Law and Ethics as Guides.* New York and Oxford: Oxford University Press.

Arena, J.F., and Lubs, H.A. 1991. Computerized approach to X-linked mental retardation syndromes. *American Journal of Medical Genetics* 38: 190–9.

Arthur D. Little, Inc. 1992. *Telecommunications: Can It Help Solve America's Health Care Problems?* Cambridge, Mass.: Arthur D. Little.

Barhyte, D.Y. 1987. Ethical issues in automating nursing personnel data. *Computers in Nursing* 5(5): 171–4.

Bartlett, E.E. 1994. Computers can thwart medical malpractice claims. *Risk Management,* June: 67–71.

Bashir, S.A., and Duffy, S.W. 1995. Correction of risk estimates for measurement error in epidemiology. *Methods of Information in Medicine* 34: 503–10.

Beauchamp, T.L., and Childress, J.F. 1994. *Principles of Biomedical Ethics,* 4th ed. New York: Oxford University Press.

Benjamin, M., and Curtis, J. 1992. *Ethics in Nursing,* 3rd ed. New York: Oxford University Press.

Betts, M. 1990. Users plot open systems revolt. *Computerdata* 15(8):10.

Bogner, M.S. ed. 1994. *Human Error in Medicine.* Hillsdale, N.J.: Lawrence Erlbaum Associates.

Boguski, M.S. 1995. Hunting for genes in computer data bases. *New England Journal of Medicine* 333: 645–7.

Boon, M.E., and Kok, L.P. 1993. Neural network processing can provide means to catch errors that slip through human screening of Pap smears. *Diagnostic Cytopathology* 9: 411–16.

Borzo, G. 1995. Physicians who computerize save on liability premiums. *American Medical News,* February 6: 5.

Bosk, C.L. 1979. *Forgive and Remember: Managing Medical Failure.* Chicago: University of Chicago Press.

Brooks, J.H.J., Renz, K.K., Kattoua, S., White, S.E., Richardson, S.L., and Delgigante, J. 1993. Linking environmental and health care databases: assessing the health effects of environmental pollutants. *International Journal of Biomedical Computing* 32: 279–88.

Brown, G.S., and Kornmayer, K. 1996. Expert systems restructure managed care practice: implementation and ethics. *Behavioral Healthcare Tomorrow* 5(1): 31–4.

Buhle, L.E., Goldwein, J.W., and Benjamin, I. 1994. OncoLink: a multimedia oncology information resource on the Internet. In *Proceedings of the Eighteenth Annual Symposium on Computer Applications in Medical Care,* ed. J.G. Ozbolt, pp. 103–7. Philadelphia: Hanley & Belfus.

Bulkeley, W.M. 1995. E-mail medicine: untested treatments, cures find stronghold on on-line services. *Wall Street Journal,* February 27: A1, A9.

Callahan D. 1994. Bioethics: private choice and common good. *Hastings Center Report* 24(3): 28–31.

Clouser, K.D., and Gert, B. 1990. A critique of principlism. *Journal of Medicine and Philosophy* 15: 219–36.

Colby, K.M. 1986. Ethics of computer assisted psychotherapy. *Professional Psychology: Research & Practice* 19: 286–9.

Coughlin, S.C. 1996. Ethically optimized study designs in epidemiology. In *Ethics and Epidemiology,* ed. S.C. Coughlin and T.L. Beauchamp, pp. 145–55. New York: Oxford University Press.

Coughlin, S.C., and Beauchamp, T.L. eds. 1996. *Ethics and Epidemiology.* New York: Oxford University Press.

Davies, B.L. 1996. A discussion of safety issues for medical robots. In *Computer-Integrated Surgery: Technology and Clinical Applications,* ed. R.H. Taylor, S. Lavallée, G.C. Burdea, and R. Mösges, pp. 287–96. Cambridge, Mass.: MIT Press.

de Dombal, F.T. 1987. Ethical considerations concerning computers in medicine in the 1980s. *Journal of Medical Ethics* 13: 179–84.

Delaplain, C.B., Lindborg, C.E., Norton, S.A., and Hastings, J.E. 1993. Tripler pioneers telemedicine across the Pacific. *Hawaii Medical Journal* 52: 338–9.

DeMaeseneer, J., and Beolchi, L. 1995. *Telematics in Primary Care in Europe.* Washington, D.C., IOS Press.

Denning, D.E., and Lin, H.S. eds. 1994. *Rights and Responsibilities of Participants in Networked Communities.* Washington, D.C.: National Academy Press.

Derr, J. 1994. Teaching ethical practice in statistics. *Amstat News,* May: 13–14.

Derse, A.R., and Krogull, S.R. 1994. The Bioethics Online Service – an implementation of a bioethics database and information resource. In *Proceedings, Eighteenth Annual Symposium on Computer Applications in Medical Care,* ed. J.G. Ozbolt, pp. 354–7. Philadelphia: Hanley & Belfus.

Dexter, P.R., Gramelspacher, G.P., Wolinsky, F.D., Zhou, X.H., and Tierney, W.M. 1996. Computer reminders, discussions of end-of-life care, and completion of advance directives. Paper presented at Annual Meeting of the Society of General Internal Medicine.

Dickson, D. 1995. Open access to sequence data "will boost hunt for breast cancer gene." *Nature* 378: 425.

Dworkin, R.M. 1977. *Taking Rights Seriously.* Cambridge, Mass.: Harvard University Press.

Ferguson. T. 1995. *Health Online: How to Go Online to Find Health Information, Support Systems, and Self-Help Communities in Cyberspace.* Reading, Mass.: Addison-Wesley.

Ferguson, E.W., Doarn, C.R., Scott, J.C. 1995. Survey of global telemedicine. *Journal of Medical Systems* 19: 35–46.

Food and Drug Administration. 1996. Meeting Summary: FDA CADx Open Public Workshop. Rockville, Md.: Food and Drug Administation (document available on the World Wide Web at http://www.fda.gov/cdrh/cadxmin. html).

Ford, B.D. 1993. Ethical and professional issues in computer assisted therapy. *Computers in Human Behavior* 9: 387–400.

Fox, J. 1993. Decision-support systems as safety-critical components: towards a safety culture for medical informatics. *Methods of Information in Medicine* 32: 345–8.

Frame, P.S., Zimmer, J.G., Werth, P.L., Hall, W.J., and Eberly, S.W. 1994. Computer-based vs manual health maintenance tracking. *Archives of Family Medicine* 3:581–8.

Frankel, M.S., and Teich, A. eds. 1994. *The Genetic Frontier: Ethics, Law, and Policy.* Washington, D.C.: American Association for the Advancement of Science.

Franken, E.A., Berbaum, K.S., Smith, W.L., Chang, P., Driscoll, C., and Bergus, G. 1992. Teleradiology for consultation between practitioners and radiologists. In *Extended Clinical Consulting by Hospital Computer Networks*, Annals of the New York Academy of Sciences, vol. 670, ed. D.F. Parsons, C.M. Fleischer, and R.A. Greenes, pp. 277–80. New York: New York Academy of Sciences.

Friedman, C.P., and Dev, P. 1996. Education and informatics: it's time to join forces. *Journal of the American Medical Informatics Association* 3: 184–5.

Gamerman, G.E. 1992. FDA regulation of biomedical software. In *Proceedings of the Sixteenth Annual Symposium on Computer Applications in Medical Care*, ed. M.E. Frisse, pp. 745–9. New York: McGraw-Hill.

Gert, B. 1989. *Morality: A New Justification of the Moral Rules.* New York: Oxford University Press.

Gilbert, S. 1996. On-line health tips offer vast mountains of gems and junk. *New York Times*, April 4: B8, National Edition.

Glowniak, J.V., and Bushway, M.K. 1994. Computer networks as a medical resource: accessing and using the Internet. *Journal of the American Medical Association* 271: 1934–9.

Goodman, K.W. 1992. Electronic roundtables for medical ethics. *Kennedy Institute of Ethics Journal* 2: 233–51.

Goodman, K.W. 1993. Monitoring ethics. *Physicians and Computers* 10 (March): 10–12.

Goodman, K.W. 1996a. Ethical Issues in Telemedicine. Working Papers in

Ethics and Policy. Miami: University of Miami Forum for Bioethics and Philosophy.

Goodman, K.W. 1996b. Ethics, genomics and information retrieval. *Computers in Biology and Medicine* 26: 223–9.

Goodman, K.W. 1996c. Machine Translation and Informed Consent. Working Papers in Ethics and Policy. Miami: University of Miami Forum for Bioethics and Philosophy.

Goodman, K.W., and Prineas, R.J. 1996. Toward an ethics curriculum in epidemiology. In *Ethics and Epidemiology*, ed. S. Coughlin and T. Beauchamp, pp. 290–303. New York: Oxford University Press.

Gorovitz, S., and MacIntyre, A. 1976. Toward a theory of medical fallibility. *Journal of Medicine and Philosophy* 1: 51–71.

Gostin, L. 1991. Ethical principles for the conduct of human subject research: population-based research and ethics. *Law, Medicine and Health Care* 19: 191–201.

Gunby, P. 1995. International electronic link solves medical puzzle. *Journal of the American Medical Association* 274: 1750.

Hamilton, R.A. 1995. FDA examining computer diagnosis. *FDA Consumer* 29(7): 20–4.

Hammond, W.E. 1995. The status of healthcare standards in the United States. *International Journal of Biomedical Computing* 39: 87–92.

Heathfield, H.A., and Wyatt, J.C. 1995. The road to professionalism in medical informatics: a proposal for debate. *Methods of Information in Medicine* 34: 426–33.

Hilgartner, S. 1995. Biomolecular databases. *Science Communication* 17:240–63.

Holmes, H.B., and Purdy, L.M. eds. 1992. *Feminist Perspectives in Medical Ethics*. Bloomington: Indiana University Press.

Jonsen, A.R., and Toulmin, S.E. 1988. *The Abuse of Casuistry*. Berkeley: University of California Press.

Kaltenborn, K.-F., and Rienhoff, O. 1993. Virtual reality in medicine. *Methods of Information in Medicine* 32: 407–17.

Kluge, W.-H. W. 1993. Advanced patient records: some ethical and legal considerations touching medical information space. *Methods of Information in Medicine* 32: 95–103.

Lamberg, L. 1996. Patients go on-line for support. *American Medical News* 39(13), April 1: 10–12, 15.

Lamson, R.J. 1995. Virtual therapy: the treatment of phobias in cyberspace. *Behavioral Healthcare Tomorrow* 4(1): 51–3.

Lancet. 1991. Being and believing: ethics of virtual reality (editorial). *Lancet* 338: 283–4.

LaPorte, R.E. 1994. Standards for information systems in the global health network. *Lancet* 344: 1640–1.

LaPorte, R.E., Akazawa, S., Hellmonds, P., Boostrom, E., Gamboa, C., Gooch, T., Hussain, F., Libman, I., Marler, E., Roko, K., Sauer, F., and Tajima, N. 1994. Global public health and the Information Superhighway. *British Medical Journal* 308:1651–2.

Leape, L.L. 1994. Error in medicine. *Journal of the American Medical Association* 272: 1851–7.

Lessenberry, J. 1996. Many turning to Internet for aid with suicide. *New York Times*, July 15: A6, National Edition.

Lipson, L. 1995. *State Initiatives to Promote Telemedicine*. Washington, D.C.: Intergovernmental Health Policy Project, George Washington University.

Lock, M. 1994. Interrogating the human diversity genome project. *Social Science and Medicine* 39: 603–6.

Loewy, E.H. 1995. Care ethics: a concept in search of a framework. *Cambridge Quarterly of Healthcare Ethics* 4: 56–63.

Ludemann, P. 1994. Mid-term report on the Arden Syntax in a clinical event monitor. *Computers in Biology and Medicine* 24: 377–83.

MacIntyre, A.C. 1981. *After Virtue: A Study in Moral Theory.* Notre Dame, Ind.: Notre Dame University Press.

Mango, L.J. 1994. Computer-assisted cervical cancer screening using neural networks. *Cancer Letters* 77: 155–62.

McGowan, J., Evans, J., and Michl, K. 1995. Networking a need: a cost-effective approach to statewide health information delivery. In *Proceedings of the Nineteenth Annual Symposium on Computer Applications in Medical Care,* ed. R.M. Gardner, pp. 571–5. Philadelphia: Hanley & Belfus.

Mercier, A.M. 1990. Expert system standards on the way? *Computerdata* 15(8): 10, 13.

Merril, J.R. 1994. The future of virtual reality, medicine, and the Information Superhighway. *Heuristics* 7 (Spring): 33–5.

Miller, P.L., Nadkarni, P.M., Kidd, K.K., Cheung, K., Ward, D., Banks, A., Bray-Ward, P., Cupelli, L. Herdman, V., Marondel, I., Montgomery, K., Renault, B., Yoon, S.-J., Krauter, K.S., and Kucherlapati, R. 1995. Internet-based support for bioscience research: a collaborative genome center for human chromosome 12. *Journal of the American Medical Informatics Association* 2: 351–64.

Miller, R.A., Schaffner, K.F., and Meisel, A. 1985. Ethical and legal issues related to the use of computer programs in clinical medicine. *Annals of Internal Medicine* 102: 529–36.

Moor, J.H. 1979. Are there decisions computers should never make? *Nature and System* 1: 217–29.

Norton, S.A., Lindborg, E.C., and Delaplain, C.B. 1993. Consent and privacy in telemedicine. *Hawaii Medical Journal* 52:340–1.

Paget, M.A. 1988. *The Unity of Mistakes: A Phenomenological Interpretation of Medical Work.* Philadelphia: Temple University Press.

Parsons, D.F., Fleischer, C.M., and Greenes, R.A. eds. 1992. *Extended Clinical Consulting by Hospital Computer Networks,* Annals of the New York Academy of Sciences, vol. 670. New York: New York Academy of Sciences.

Pellegrino, E.D., and Thomasma, D.C. 1993. *The Virtues in Medical Practice.* New York: Oxford University Press.

Pemble, K.R. 1994. Regional health information networks: the Wisconsin Health Information Network, a case study. In *Proceedings of the Eighteenth Annual Symposium on Computer Applications in Medical Care,* ed. J.G. Ozbolt, pp. 401–5. Philadelphia: Hanley & Belfus.

Perednia, D.A., Gaines, J.A., and Butruille, T.W. 1995. Comparison of the clinical informativeness of photographs and digital imaging media with multiple-choice receiver operating characteristic analysis. *Archives of Dermatology* 131: 292–7.

Pickering, G.W. 1955. Disorders of contemporary society and their impact on medicine. *Annals of Internal Medicine* 43: 919–29.

Preston, J. 1994. *The Telemedicine Handbook: Improving Health Care with Interactive Video,* 2nd ed. Austin, Tex.: Telemedical Interactive Consultative Services.

Rawls, J. 1971. *A Theory of Justice.* Cambridge, Mass.: Harvard University Press.

Roberts, L. 1992. How to sample the world's genetic diversity. *Science* 257: 1204–5.

Sadegh-Zadeh, K. 1989. Machine over mind. *Artificial Intelligence in Medicine* 1: 3–10.

Safran, C., and Chute, C.G. 1995. Exploration and exploitation of clinical databases. *International Journal of Biomedical Computing* 39: 151–6.

Salaman, J.R., Griffin, P.J.A., Ross, W., and Haines, J. 1994. Lifeline Wales: experience with a computerised kidney donor registry. *British Medical Journal* 308: 30–1.

Sieghart, P., and Dawson, J. 1987. Computer-aided medical ethics. *Journal of Medical Ethics* 13(4): 185–8.

Smoyak, S.A. 1986. High tech/high touch. *Nursing Success Today* 3 (11): 8–16.

Szolovits, P. 1995. Uncertainty and decisions in medical informatics. *Methods of Information in Medicine* 34: 111–21.

Szolovits, P., and Pauker, S.G. 1979. Computers and clinical decision making: whether, how much, and for whom? *Proceedings of the IEEE* 67: 1224–6.

Taylor, R.H., Lavallée, S., Burdea, G.C., and Mösges, R. eds. 1996. *Computer-Integrated Surgery: Technology and Clinical Applications.* Cambridge, Mass.: MIT Press.

Thacker, S.B., and Stroup, D.F. 1994. Future directions for comprehensive public health surveillance and health information systems in the United States. *American Journal of Epidemiology* 140: 383–97.

Waldrop, M.M. 1995. On-line archives let biologists interrogate the genome. *Science* 269:1356–8.

Weizenbaum, J. 1976. *Computer Power and Human Reason: From Judgment to Calculation.* Boston: Freeman.

Whalley, L.J. 1995. Ethical issues in the application of virtual reality to medicine. *Computers in Biology and Medicine* 25:107–14.

Whitney, C.R. 1996. In France, national health care meets a Gallic version of H.M.O. *New York Times*, April 25: A6, National Edition.

Wikler, D. 1989. Equity, efficacy, and the point system for transplant recipient selection. *Transplantation Proceedings* 21: 3437–9.

Wilkins, G. 1994. Mental health informatics. In *Computers in Mental Health,* vol. 1, ed. T.B.Üstün, pp. 16–23. Edinburgh: Churchill Livingstone and the World Health Organization.

Williams, N. 1995. Europe opens institute to deal with gene data deluge. *Science* 269: 630.

Wolkon, G.H., and Lyon, M. 1986. Ethical issues in computerized mental health data systems. *Hospital & Community Psychiatry* 37 (1): 11–12, 16.

Woolery, L.K. 1990. Professional standards and ethical dilemmas in nursing information systems. *Journal of Nursing Administration* 20 (10): 50–3.

2

Medical informatics and human values

TERRELL WARD BYNUM AND JOHN L. FODOR

Telling right from wrong often requires appeal to a set of values. Some values are general or global, and they range across the spectrum of human endeavor. Identifying and ranking such values, and being clear about their conflicts and exceptions, is an important philosophical undertaking. Other values are particular or local. They may be special cases of the general values. So when "freedom from pain" is offered in the essay by Professors Bynum and Fodor as a *medical* value, it is conceptually linked to freedom, a general value. Local values apply within and often among different human actions: law, medicine, engineering, journalism, computing, education, business, and so forth. To be consistent, a commitment to a value in any of these domains should not contradict global values. To be sure, tension between and among local and global values is the stuff of exciting debate in applied ethics. And sometimes a particular local value will point to *consequences* that are at odds with a general value. Debates over these tensions likewise inform the burgeoning literature in applied or professional ethics. In this chapter, Bynum and Fodor apply the seminal work of James H. Moor in an analysis of the values that apply in the health professions. What emerges is a straightforward perspective on the way to think about advancing health computing while paying homage to those values.

1 – A robot may not injure a human being, or, through inaction, allow a human being to come to harm.
2 – A robot must obey the orders given it by human beings except where such orders would conflict with the First Law.
3 – A robot must protect its own existence as long as such protection does not conflict with the First or Second Law.
(*The Three Laws of Robotics,* Handbook of Robotics, *56th Edition, 2058 A.D.* [Asimov 1950])

We would like to acknowledge our indebtedness to the writings of James H. Moor of Dartmouth College, especially his prize-winning essay "What Is Computer Ethics?" (Moor 1985), and his classic article "Are There Decisions Computers Should Never Make?" (Moor 1979).

The computer revolution and computer ethics

If this were an ideal world, technology would have only good effects on the things we value. But of course the world is not ideal, and technology has both positive and negative effects. The more powerful the technology, the more profound are the effects. For this reason, genuine revolutions in technology – like the Agricultural or the Industrial revolutions – bring about major benefits for human beings: longer lives, food for the hungry, relief from heavy labor, rapid and comfortable transportation, to cite just a few examples. But the very same revolutionary technology also brings about or is impotent against monumental problems: Consider over-population, pollution, and weapons of mass destruction.

Truly revolutionary technology, then, has a major impact on the things people value most. As philosophers, we can argue at great length about the nature, significance, and relative importance of human values such as health, security, freedom, and knowledge. Yet as human beings, we cherish these values and try to advance them. Consequently, any technology that seriously affects our values is of central importance to us.

The most recent technological revolution is the Computer Revolution. No longer are "computers" simply giant machines confined to research laboratories or corporate accounting offices. They now appear as laptop portables and are used in hearing aids, home appliances, medical equipment, military hardware, factory assembly lines, automobiles, satellites, and on and on.

The Computer Revolution will likely become the biggest and most profound technological revolution of all. This is mostly because of the "logical malleability" of computers. As James Moor explains:

> The essence of the Computer Revolution is found in the nature of the computer itself. What is revolutionary about computers is *logical malleability*. . . . The logic of computers can be massaged and shaped in endless ways through changes in hardware and software. Just as the power of a steam engine was a raw resource of the Industrial Revolution, so the logic of a computer is a raw resource of the Computer Revolution. Because logic applies everywhere, the potential applications of computer technology appear limitless. The computer is the nearest thing we have to a universal tool. Indeed, the limits of computers are largely the limits of our own creativity (Moor 1985: 269).

Computer technology is not exempt from the tendency of all technology to have both positive and negative effects. We are all familiar with impressive, positive "breakthroughs" made possible by computer technology: desktop publishing, worldwide networking, CAT scans, photographs from distant planets, and so forth. Regrettably, we are just as familiar with news reports about computer risks and harms: "hackers" who invade people's privacy, computer-aided bank robbery, malfunctions that cause terrible accidents, etc. To study the positive and negative impacts of computer technology, a new branch of applied ethics – *computer ethics* – has emerged during the past two decades. This new field of research

> examines the impact of computing and information technology upon human values, using concepts, theories and procedures from philosophy, sociology, law, psychology, and so on. Practitioners of . . . computer ethics – whether they are philosophers, computer scientists, social scientists, public policy makers, or whatever – all have the same goal: To integrate computing technology and human values in such a way that the technology advances and protects human values, rather than doing damage to them (Bynum 1992: 16).

During the past several years, researchers in computer ethics have focused for the most part upon a few "standard" topics like privacy, security, software ownership, responsibility for malfunctions, computer-caused problems in the workplace, and replacement and displacement of human beings by computerized devices (Bynum 1985; Johnson 1994; Perrolle 1987). Some concerns that have made international headlines include possible invasions of privacy resulting from use of huge databases (Bynum, Maner, and Fodor 1992b), computer viruses that "crash" a system or do other harm (Spafford, Heaphy, and Ferbrache 1989), and "hackers" who compromise national security (Neumann 1995).

Much like computing in general, medical computing has both positive and negative consequences. For example, on the positive side, consider computer-assisted technology for persons with disabilities, technology such as computerized artificial limbs, pacemakers, inner-ear implants, and electronic voice generators (Bynum, Maner, and Fodor 1992a). On the negative side, consider the Therac-25 case in which patients were killed or maimed by an X-ray machine with faulty software (Leveson and Turner 1993). These examples and many more clearly demonstrate that medical computing affects broad human values, such as freedom and security.

In addition to human values in general, there are certain specific ones that people usually associate with medicine. These include, for example, health, freedom from pain, and access to care. To preserve and advance these and related values, medical professionals perform a wide variety of tasks. These include:

• Information gathering and data acquisition (interviews, filling out forms, observations, examinations, tests)

- Recordkeeping and updating
- Educating patients, their families, and caregivers
- Diagnosis
- Prognosis
- Prescription of therapy
- Delivery of therapy (drugs, bodily manipulations, surgery, prostheses, psychological counseling)
- Monitoring (interviews, observations and examinations, tests, assessment of progress)
- Adjustment of therapy
- Daily physical support and care (hygiene, nutrition, etc.)
- Psychological support and sympathy

Virtually every one of these tasks is now aided in one way or another by computers. Obvious examples include databases of patient histories, electronic thermometers, monitors that alert hospital staff to life-threatening emergencies, CAT scans, computer-aided laser surgery. Even a task like patient education – which used not to be considered a candidate for computer assistance – can now be undertaken by computerized instructional materials such as CD-ROMs (e.g., Veenstra and Gluck 1991) and patient information sheets that can be downloaded from the World Wide Web. Computer technology is rapidly becoming ubiquitous in health care.

Computers or health professionals?

The examples cited here make it clear that computerized devices are used in a variety of ways to aid medical professionals in the performance of their duties. But besides aiding humans, *is it possible for computers to replace human beings and perform medical and nursing tasks by themselves?* For many "routine" tasks, the answer is, yes, they can – indeed, they already do. For example, computerized devices in intensive care units monitor and record a patient's temperature, blood pressure, and heart rate while making this information available to staff members or to other computers. In addition, a wide variety of laboratory tests that once were conducted by human technicians now are routinely performed by computerized machines. And for certain ailments, computerized devices administer medication directly into the patient.

A recent example of how computers are replacing humans in health care is the service being tested by the Harvard Community Health Plan, a health maintenance organization in Massachusetts. To get medical advice

36   *Terrell Ward Bynum and John L. Fodor*

at home, patients dial a toll-free telephone number and interact with a computer. After the patient provides a computer with some answers to questions about symptoms, health history, and so on, the computer prescribes a home remedy, such as gargling with salt water or taking a pain reliever; or it arranges for a physician or nurse to call the patient; or it gives the patient an appointment at the clinic (Freudenheim 1991).

So, increasingly, computers are replacing human beings in the delivery of medical services. Whether or not a particular medical task can be performed by a computer is an empirical question; that is, it is not possible to know the answer in advance, or without testing. One must conduct experiments and compare the computer's track record to that of relevant medical professionals. And, of course, as computer technology improves, tasks that once were impossible for computers to perform may eventually become computerized.

Certain medical roles are bound to be harder for computers to fulfill than others. For example, tasks which normally are thought to require "judgment" or "clinical intuition" or "human sympathy and compassion" may prove to be the hardest ones for computers to perform successfully. These include diagnosis, prognosis, prescription of therapy, and psychological counseling (see the discussion in Chapter 6).

Consider diagnosis, for example. The sophistication and complexity of medical diagnosis and the difficult challenge of trying to computerize it are described by Randolph Miller in his keystone article, "Why the Standard View Is Standard":

Diagnosis is an "art" because it represents a sequence of interdependent, often highly individualized processes: elicitation of initial patient data; integration of the data into plausible scenarios regarding known disease processes; evaluating and refining of diagnostic hypotheses through selective elicitation of additional patient information; initiation of therapy at appropriate points in time (including before a diagnosis is established); and evaluation of the effect of both the illness and the therapy on the patient over time (Miller 1990: 584; also see Mazoué 1990).

Another very challenging health-related task that is difficult to computerize is psychological counseling. Nevertheless, even this skill can be aided by computerized devices, for example, by ones that conduct preliminary interviews or provide reassuring information and instruction.

Even the early, and by today's standards simplistic, "psychotherapy" computer program ELIZA (Weizenbaum 1976) provided psychological comfort to some of the people who used it. And they were computer-literate students and faculty members who knew how the program worked!

As Sherry Turkle explains: "With full knowledge that the program could not empathize with them, they confided in it, and wanted to be alone with it" (Turkle 1984: 39). In an era of complex simulations and virtual reality, it is possible to give computers human-like faces and voices. Current and future "electronic counselors" will continue to have a much stronger effect upon people than ELIZA (Illovsky 1994). Weizenbaum himself strongly objected to any serious suggestion that ELIZA-like "psychotherapy" programs should actually be used with patients. (We return to this issue below.)

Harm caused by medical computing

Time will tell whether or not computers will ever be able to perform tasks which now require human "judgment," "intuition," and "sympathy." In the meantime, it is clear that the effects of medical computing, so far, have been very positive: Many lives have been saved, many diseases cured, many pains relieved. Still, there are risks from any medical procedure, and sometimes there are terrible consequences (see Snapper's account of responsibility in Chapter 3). Medical computing has, on occasion, caused serious harm. Perhaps the best-known example is that of the Therac-25. In other cases, people have died when their pacemakers were reprogrammed by antitheft equipment in stores, and an infusion pump for insulin delivered medication at the wrong rates (Forester and Morrison 1990).

Should unhappy cases like these cause the medical profession to avoid computers? Certainly not! All medical procedures have risks, and some, despite our best intentions, yield harmful results. The underlying question is not whether there are risks involved in using computers but rather whether computers enhance our commitment to human values and, hence, our ability to minimize pain and preserve human life and health. Where computers have a better track record than humans, or where they work better for record keeping, research, etc., it would be unethical not to use them, unless costs are prohibitive or patients can choose to opt out, and do so.

Are there tasks computers should not perform?

Computers do help us to fulfill the goals of medicine. And, at least in certain narrowly defined domains, they even outperform and replace physicians, nurses, and other health professionals. And because medical computing is still in its infancy, this trend is likely to continue and accelerate. In the coming years we can expect more and more health-related tasks to be performed by computers, altering (perhaps, in the *very* long run, even eliminating) the roles of physicians, nurses, laboratory technicians, counselors, and others.

It is important, therefore, for the health professions – and indeed for society in general – to explore answers to a key question: *Are there health-related tasks that computers should never be permitted to perform?*

In his book, *Computer Power and Human Reason*, Joseph Weizenbaum argues that it would be immoral – indeed "madness" – to allow computers to make psychiatric judgments. He states, "What could be more obvious than the fact that, whatever intelligence a computer can muster, however it may be acquired, it must always and necessarily be absolutely alien to any and all authentic human concerns" (Weizenbaum 1976: 226). However, in response, Moor points out that it is an *empirical* question whether or not computers will ever be good counselors. He notes: "Empirically this may never happen, but it is not a necessary truth that it will not" (Moor 1979: 226).

Is there *any* medical task, then, that we know in advance computers should never perform? Two suggestions come to mind:

(1) Computers should never perform any medical task that a human wishes to perform.
(2) Computers should never perform any medical task that humans can perform more competently. (See Moor 1979 for closely related principles, which he calls "Dubious Maxims.")

At first sight, these dictums seem undeniably true. For, under most circumstances, following them will indeed advance the basic values of medicine. Each can serve as a "rule of thumb" which is normally followed. Nevertheless, strictly speaking, *each is false*, because we can find exceptions to them.

Consider the first dictum. Imagine a patient who needs a medical procedure that computers can perform better than humans (for example, computer-guided shaping of bones to receive artificial joints or other parts, or computer-controlled laser eye surgery). If the patient's physician performs the procedure anyway, knowing that computer-guided shaping is a superior procedure, he or she would be providing inferior medical care. This would not be in the best interest of the patient and would therefore be unethical. (For these examples we assume that relevant costs are commensurate.)

The second dictum suffers a similar fate: Normally, if humans can outperform computers in a given medical task, then humans should get the job. However, in certain very dangerous settings – such as outer space or on a battlefield – it may be ethically better to use computers and thereby spare humans exposure to extreme danger. In a major nuclear accident, for example, where injured people are inside a radioactive building, medical robots might be sent in to provide care for the sick, even though human physicians could provide better medical care. (Compare the point made by Sheridan and Thompson 1994, who suggest that "teleoperators" might be used to tend patients with highly contagious diseases or during acute psychotic episodes, thus protecting human caregivers, or to attend to severely immunocompromised patients, thus protecting the *patients* from provider-borne contagion.)

Both of our suggested dictums, then, while they can indeed serve as useful "rules of thumb," have exceptions. Where does this leave us? Is there nothing in medicine that humans should reserve to themselves? The answer becomes clear when we think of the ultimate human values upon which medicine rests: values such as life, health, and freedom from pain. Choosing the fundamental goals of medicine and setting priorities among them are tasks that we should never turn over to a computer (Moor 1979). We certainly do not want computers to decide that these values are unimportant – or that they should be sacrificed to values that a computer might choose for us.

Isaac Asimov's once fanciful "laws of robotics" work as a literary device to elicit a variety of interesting man-machine tensions. That the tensions are nontrivial, usually involving life and or death, is noteworthy. The way we resolve tensions in the real world, with or without robots or intelligent medical machines, is by appeal to shared or core values. It is not just that we will not allow computers to identify our values, but that we also will not let them act in conflict with the values we have already embraced. One might think of this as drawing a line in the silicon.

Future prospects

What are some prospects for the future if our analysis is correct? We began this chapter by noting that computer technology has both positive and negative effects. Let us therefore itemize particulars that embody both possibilities.

Positive possibilities

Greater access. Given the existence of worldwide computer networks, and the likes of the U.S. and European plans for "National Information

Infrastructures," the example of the Harvard Community Health Plan may be magnified dramatically in just a few years. Automated medical services are already available "on-line" or at clinics with a minimal human staff, providing health services to rural and economically depressed areas, isolated outposts, and other places where health care is normally scarce. Eventually, more and more health care will be provided "over the net" in the comfort of one's own home.

Improved quality. As computers become better tools for human decision making, this is one of the benefits reasonably to be expected.

Affordability. If market forces act on medical computers as they have on pocket calculators, personal computers, and indeed nearly all computing technology, we could see a tremendous reduction in cost. This could help reduce overall health expenditures and keep them more in line with inflation.

Equity. At present (mid-late 1990s), more than 260 million people around the world have no access to health care; in the United States, the largest industrialized country without a national health plan, 40 million people have no health insurance, and 50 million more are underinsured. Increased affordability and accessibility could dramatically eliminate this enormous injustice in one medical care delivery system, especially if government regulations require that the poor gain fair access to the "Information Superhighway."

Negative possibilities

Skill degradation. It has been suggested that increased reliance on computerized systems might cause humans to lose certain skills best not lost (see the discussion in Chapter 6). The likelihood and extent of this serious possibility are extraordinarily difficult to determine.

Erosion of traditionally useful relationships. It is commonplace to note the therapeutic value of physician-, nurse-, therapist-, and other provider-patient relationships. If reliance on computers damages or eliminates these relationships without providing countervailing benefits, the effect would be most unfortunate (again see the discussion in Chapter 6).

Overpopulation. If affordable, high-quality medical care becomes available throughout the world, many more lives will be saved and prolonged. That would indeed be a boon to humanity. Still, as a result of this achievement, some regions of the world could experience overpopulation, or worse overpopulation, with all its attendant problems of scarcity and political instability.

Greed. It is at least conceivable that vested interests in the medical industry might resist the development and widespread use of inexpensive high-quality medical computing devices, intending to keep medical costs and profits high. If high-quality medical computing evolves in the same way as other health technologies, and is controlled by a monopoly or cartel or profiteers, it is bound to be extremely expensive – unless, of course, society intervenes to keep prices at affordable levels.

Conclusion: Accentuate the positive

In this chapter we make a number of observations and advance several claims. Much of this was, we suggest, simply to point out the obvious: We observed that computer technology is becoming ubiquitous in medicine, mentioned that computerized devices now perform a number of tasks that once were performed by medical professionals, and noted that, like technology in general, medical computing has both positive and negative effects upon the things we value.

In trying to decide what computers should not be permitted to do, we argued that issues about where and how to use computers in medicine are, for the most part, empirical. They can be answered only by comparing human track records with those of computers to see which ones advance our fundamental values better. However, choosing and ranking those fundamental values themselves are tasks that we should reserve for human beings and deny to computers.

Since fundamental human values are involved, and since computers are performing more and more health-related tasks, it is apparent that bioethicists need to pay attention to these developments. They should monitor health computing to ensure that it advances human values, and they should call our attention to cases where it does not.

Finally, society should recognize the tremendous potential of this technology to affect our deepest values. We must ensure that medical computing develops in such a way that its positive effects are maximized and its negative effects are minimized.

References

Asimov, I. 1950. *I, Robot.* Greenwich, Conn.: Fawcett Crest.

Bynum, T.W. ed. 1985. *Computers and Ethics.* Oxford: Blackwell. (Published as the October 1985 issue of the journal *Metaphilosophy.*)

Bynum, T.W. 1992. Human values and the computer science curriculum. In *Teaching Computing and Human Values,* ed. T.W. Bynum, W. Maner, and J.L. Fodor, pp. 15–34. New Haven, Conn.: Research Center on Computing & Society, Southern Connecticut State University.

Bynum, T.W., Maner, W., and Fodor, J.L., eds. 1992a. *Equity and Access to Computing Resources*: New Haven, Conn.: Research Center on Computing & Society, Southern Connecticut State University.

Bynum, T.W., Maner, W., and Fodor, J.L., eds. 1992b. *Computing and Privacy.* New Haven, Conn.: Research Center on Computing & Society, Southern Connecticut State University.

Forester, T., and Morrison, P. 1990. *Computer Ethics: Cautionary Tales and Ethical Dilemmas in Computing.* Cambridge, Mass.: MIT Press.

Freudenheim, M. 1991. Computer says take two aspirin. *New York Times,* June 25: D2, New York Edition.

Illovsky, M.E. 1994. Counseling, artificial intelligence, and expert systems. *Simulation & Gaming* 25: 88–98.

Johnson, D.G. 1994. *Computer Ethics,* 2nd ed. Englewood Cliffs, N.J.: Prentice-Hall.

Leveson, N., and Turner, C. 1993. An investigation of the Therac-25 accidents. *Computer* 26: 18–41.

Mazoué, J.G. 1990. Diagnosis without doctors. *Journal of Medicine and Philosophy* 15: 559–79.

Miller, R.A. 1990. Why the standard view is standard: people, not machines, understand patients' problems. *Journal of Medicine and Philosophy* 15: 581–91.

Moor, J.H. 1979. Are there decisions computers should never make? *Nature and System* 1: 217–229.

Moor, J.H. 1985. What is computer ethics? In *Computers and Ethics,* ed. T.W. Bynum, pp. 266–75. Oxford: Blackwell.

Neumann, P.G. 1995. *Computer-Related Risks.* New York: ACM Press.

Perrolle, J.A. 1987. *Computers and Social Change: Information, Property and Power.* Belmont, Calif.: Wadsworth.

Sheridan, T.B., and Thompson, J.M. 1994. People versus computers in medicine. In *Human Error in Medicine,* ed. M.S. Bogner, pp.141–58. Hillsdale, N.J.: Lawrence Erlbaum Associates.

Spafford, E.H., Heaphy, K.A., and Ferbrache, D.J. 1989. *Computer Viruses.* Arlington, Va.: ADAPSO.

Turkle, S. 1984. *The Second Self.* New York: Simon & Schuster.

Veenstra, R.J., and Gluck, J.C. 1991. Access to information about AIDS. *Annals of Internal Medicine* 114: 320–4.

Weizenbaum, J. 1976. *Computer Power and Human Reason: From Judgment to Calculation.* Boston: Freeman.

3

Responsibility for computer-based decisions in health care

JOHN W. SNAPPER

When errors are made or things go wrong or decisions are beguiled, there is a very powerful and common human inclination to assess and apportion responsibility: *Who's to blame?* Whether any particular act of commission or omission is morally blameworthy is determined against a broad background of shared values and in the context of more or less deep understandings of causation and responsibility. In this chapter, Professor John W. Snapper develops his distinctive model for evaluating responsibility for computer-based medical decisions. In this model, the computer emerges as an agent that can be deemed responsible for certain kinds of errors. With the goal of promoting appropriate computer use by clinicians, Professor Snapper's distinctive analysis avoids conundrums about causes of harms, and eschews puzzles that often arise in attempting to identify foreseeable risks. Rather, it presents an argument for spreading responsibility and diversifying duty. Professor Snapper argues that appropriately attributing responsibility and duty to computers for certain actions will maximize the social goods that would follow from broader use of machines for decision support. What is increasingly clear is that legal approaches to error and liability in medical computing are inadequate in the absence of thoroughgoing conceptual and ethical analyses of responsibility, accountability, and blame.

Mechanical judgments and intelligent machines

Modern medical practice makes use of a variety of "intelligent machines" that evaluate patient conditions, help in literature searches, interpret laboratory data, monitor patients, and much more. This chapter explores options for assigning responsibility for "judgments" made by intelligent machines in patient care. It develops a line of reasoning that began more than a decade ago (Snapper 1985) and suggests that if certain criteria are met it is appropriate to assign responsibility to intelligent machines.

Consider, for instance, accountability for actions taken by a monitoring

43

system that responds to a patient's condition, but responds differently from what may be expected of an attending human physician. One issue is the sort of standards that should be applied to the machine; for example, should the machine keep itself aware of medical advances in a way analogous to the way physicians stay aware of changes in medical practice? We should also ask who should be subject to liability for failure to satisfy those standards. Would it be reasonable, for instance, for hospitals to provide malpractice insurance for expert machines, just as they do for human physicians?

The issues are not drawn from speculative fiction. At an elementary level, we often use machines to monitor and correct irregular heartbeat or abnormal blood-sugar levels for hospitalized patients. Although these "simple" machine responses hardly deserve to be viewed as human-like "judgments," the machines are performing functions that were quite recently performed by human attendants (see Moor 1979 for his touchstone discussion of what it means for computers to make decisions; for a collection of accounts of *human* responsibility in health care, see Agich 1982). As such, an assessment of machine reliability has replaced discussions of human accountability for performance in these areas of medical practice. As the machines are used in more complex situations, their responses look more and more like the expert judgments made by humans. The assessment of responsibility is becoming correspondingly more complex. We can easily imagine (and perhaps expect) sophisticated systems that monitor hospitalized patients for multiple, complex conditions, and choose from a wide range of options to perform tests and administer treatments in response to unexpected patient conditions. Significant progress has been made, for instance, toward the development of automated field hospitals that help injured soldiers when human doctors would be either at risk or unavailable (Satava 1995). At that level, the ethical assessment of a machine decision is complex indeed.

The criteria we choose for assigning responsibility for machine judgments obviously affect whether and how the machines will be used. For instance, a medical practitioner may be more willing to rely on machine judgments if he or she thereby abandons personal responsibility for those judgments. Not surprisingly, then, the law of torts has become a forum for debate over the introduction of new technologies. For instance, a well-known decision on liability for failure to perform a glaucoma test has led to our present practice wherein all optometrists routinely perform glaucoma tests on constantly upgraded equipment (Fortess and Kapp 1985; Bowers 1986). It is, moreover, a cliché of modern medicine that the concerns of malpractice insurers deeply influence medical decisions over whether to introduce new machines. As a blatant example, consider those insurers who lowered their rates to physicians who used a voice-activated machine which watches for areas of concern in emergency departments (cf. Karcz et al. 1993). This machine listens to the physicians' remarks and warns them to take special care when it hears references to medical problems that are frequently the focus of litigation. No discussion of the usefulness of expert systems can be separated from decisions on how we assign responsibility for their actions.

Harms and blame, goods and credit

Possible loci of responsibility

We should seriously consider the whole range of options for the assignment of credit and blame for machine-made medical judgments. We could assign responsibility to the operators of the machines, their owners, their manufacturers, their designers, attending physicians who rely on the machines, or, simply, no one. We may reject some of these options in the long run, but no option may be ignored simply because it is nontraditional. I take seriously, for instance, the suggestion that no one be held responsible for faulty judgment (*Lohr v Medtronic*, 56 F.3d 1335 [1995]). That is, we may legislate immunity from litigation when medical practice relies on machine judgment in certain contexts. There are good reasons both for and against this approach. As one guiding principle (among many relevant medical and legal concerns), let us assume that

Responsibility should be assigned so as to encourage the use of life-enhancing technology, when it can be shown that the technology is truly life-enhancing.

The legal reality is that injured patients often sue everyone who could be involved by any available legal theory, in the hopes that some suits will hit the target. When a machine is involved, this often includes a suit against the machine manufacturer or distributor under product liability law, which assigns strict liability for flawed machinery. "Strict liability" here means that there can be no excuse for the flaw; that is, the good faith and professionalism of the producer are irrelevant. Indeed, this is the correct legal response to harms caused by machines whose bad judgments are occasioned by improperly copied software, missing wires, or some other production flaw. In my view, the Therac-25 accidents, in which software and other errors in a radiation therapy machine contributed to a number of deaths and injuries, were due to software production and testing problems, and as such deserve to be assessed under the strict liability test for product liability (Leveson and Turner 1993; cf. the discussion in Chapter 4; also, Neumann 1995 gives a catalog of computer errors from a variety of fields and applications, including medicine). There can be no excuse for bad construction of medical equipment. (For an introductory legal discussion of how traditional negligence and product liability attribute liability to a manufacturer, see Mortimer 1989. For an early, more general discussion of responsibility, see Miller, Schaffner, and Meisel 1985; also see Chapter 6 in this book.) But this is philosophically less interesting than machines that are properly put together and yet do not respond to patient needs in the same way as would the best human doctors under similar conditions. In present legal practice, product liability might also be used to sue the manufacturer/designer in this case. But it would be an odd form of product liability, since the design of the machine must be assessed against professional standards for good designs. The appeal to "professional standards" is a serious departure from the "strict liability" that characterizes the rest of product liability law. (Leveson and Turner 1993 provide a nice discussion of the lessons learned from the Therac-25 accidents for setting professional standards for testing. Also see Nissenbaum 1996 for an analysis of accountability in computing; Gotterbarn 1995 for an account of moral responsibility in software engineering; and Siegler, Toulmin, Zimring, and Schaffner 1987 for a helpful collection of papers on bad medical outcomes, including the role of causation, and aspects of responsibility.)

Rather than trace responsibility to the machine designers, I would like to draw attention to the responsibility of physicians who defer to machine judgments. In legal practice physician liability can be separable from the manufacturer's product liability, in that separate (perhaps interconnected) suits may be directed at both. Although it is also common practice to distribute blame for patient harms by assessing the relative levels of responsibility of the blameworthy (e.g., 45 percent to the physician, 35 percent to the hospital, and 20 percent to the machine maintenance company), I will concentrate on the responsibility of physicians as if it were an entirely separate matter.

Physician liability is particularly important, as a separate issue, since this has an immediate effect on the willingness of doctors to endorse the use of expert machines. Although the medical profession has generally been very receptive to new technologies (including sophisticated computerized instruments), there is resistance to the use of computerized systems that seem to make medical decisions. Two of the reasons for this resistance are apparently

(1) *a wish to keep control over decisions that have traditionally belonged to M.D.s*

(2) *a wish to keep control over decisions for which one has responsibility*

These are separate matters. (Empirical evidence for their importance to the implementation of new medical technology is presented in Anderson and Jay 1987 and Anderson, Aydin, and Jay 1994.) Item (1) will figure prominently in our discussion below of borrowed servants, and (2) will figure in our discussion of consultancy. In each case, we will attempt to encourage acceptance of expert machines by applying reasonable criteria for accountability that ease these concerns.

Computers as agents

This chapter argues that we should assess the blame of a physician who depends on an incompetent machine just as we assess the blame of a physician who depends on human consultants and other medical agents who assist the doctor's patients. This approach suggests that the machine itself could be liable for harms, analogously to cases where liability passes from the doctor to other human medical assistants. Although this option is often overlooked because of a popular misconception that legal liability can only attach to humans, there is really nothing conceptually problematic about it. The status of a computer as the defendant in legal disputes is just a matter of legal convention. We often hold things that are not in the ordinary sense ''persons'' to be liable for certain harms. We commonly sue corporations (which we perversely call ''persons'' in this context). And in certain cases (notably maritime law), we sue material items. Lawyers call such suits *ad rem*, i.e., directed ''at the thing.'' The interesting social issue is not whether this is an option, but whether we wish to write *ad rem* laws governing harms caused by computer decisions. (In that case, we would probably also write laws demanding that hospitals insure at-risk computers against liability.) Although I do not advocate the creation of such laws, I would not be terribly surprised if, in the ever-changing world of technology and law, we do at some time institute *ad rem* suits against computers.

Let us consider as an option for assessing responsibility the idea that a computerized system for medical decisions should be viewed as an agent of the physician in charge. In legal jargon, a supervising M.D. would be the "principal" and the machine would be the "agent." I take this suggestion more seriously than the suggestion that computers be the subject of *ad rem* liability because I do not think that the agency suggestion is really all that radical. Since a principal may be vicariously liable for a harm caused by his or her agents under the doctrine of *respondeat superior* ("let the master answer"), the present suggestion is compatible with leaving liability with the physician. We may also note that since principal and agent may be "jointly and severally" liable for torts, the present suggestion is also compatible with finding the machine itself responsible. So an agency approach provides us with a way to evaluate the physician's responsibility as principal, while leaving undecided the further question of the machine's individual responsibility.

This approach views the machine agent's actions as if they are human agent actions. This is a dangerous analogy, and we must be careful not to overstate it. Even if the decision-making process itself is very similar, there are obviously important differences between machines and humans that affect how we assess responsibility. Computers do not (in any foreseeable technology) regret errors. They are not deserving of pity. They are not subject to "weakness of the will." They do not enter into agency relations by accepting pay for their services. But we must also not understate the similarity between machine and human judgment. Much of the process for assessing responsibility does not depend on the human features of the agent, only on the nature of judgment. We can, for instance, evaluate the correctness of the medical judgment of machine and human by similar standards. In each case, we can inquire into whether the agent was aware, for instance, of the patient's wishes for life-support and whether it was the agent's responsibility to seek that information actively. Defibrillation machines (which regulate heartbeat) make decisions exactly like those made by human clinicians in other contexts. More sophisticated machines make more sophisticated judgments, which can be faulty in ways similar to more sophisticated human judgment. A machine may, for instance, fail to look with sufficient depth into its data, or spend too much time looking into its data when emergency action is required, or ignore symptoms that indicate a problem outside the scope of its knowledge, or not be up-to-date on new treatments, or just be more stupid than its colleagues. These are human-like faults, and not simply cases of broken machines with sticky valves.

Procedures for analyzing harms

To view a computer as an agent directs our attention to a procedure for assessing the responsibility for computer generated harms. I consider two examples. First is the adaptation of the "borrowed servant" rule to machines for automated care. In this discussion reliance on machines is treated like reliance on hospital staff. Secondly, I consider the assignment of duties to clinicians and to computerized expert systems. In this discussion reliance on machines is treated like reliance on human medical consultants. In each case I find features of the traditional human case to be useful for the computer case.

The "borrowed servant" rule

The metaphor of the borrowed servant suggests the following sort of situation. An under-chef in my restaurant gets sick on the night of an important banquet. You send an under-chef from your restaurant to help me out. Even if this borrowed servant remains in your pay, my chef and I are responsible for harms to customers he or she poisons while working in my restaurant under our supervision. A similar view may be taken toward hospital employees (nurses, interns, medical assistants) who work under the supervision of an attending M.D. who is not a hospital employee. The hospital staff may be viewed as borrowed servants of the physician, who thereby acquires responsibility for harms caused by their poor decisions. (Note that as a theory of medical torts, this approach is both common and mildly controversial; see King 1986: chapter 6 for an introductory discussion.)

There are good reasons to view a machine that monitors and responds to patient conditions, such as envisioned in the restaurant example, as a borrowed servant, analogously to the way we view human medical agents as borrowed servants of the principal M.D.

At issue is whether the physician is responsible for decisions made (and acted upon) by the machine. In the case of a borrowed servant, the question turns upon the amount of control the M.D. has over the agent. A physician's assistant who acts while watched by the physician is clearly under the control of the doctor and is a borrowed servant (lent by the hospital that may otherwise be held accountable). In that case the physician is liable for harms resulting from the assistant's decisions. A hospital nurse who cares for that patient when the physician is not even in the hospital is, however, not under the doctor's control and is not a borrowed servant. And the physician may have no liability for the nurse's decisions. The interesting questions, of course, appear in the myriad variations on these situations where it is hard to determine whether the nurse is a borrowed servant of the physician. If, for instance, the doctor carefully selects the nurses from the hospital staff and then personally trains them on special patient needs, a nurse may become a borrowed servant and the doctor may acquire vicarious responsibility for actions taken without direct supervision. (Of course, some of these relationships in actual practice are changing as nurses acquire more direct decision-making authority and responsibility as primary care providers. The borrowed servant analogy should also be applied in the context of nursing informatics. Use of the term "servant" here is thus in no sense intended to suggest that it captures the best or most appropriate relationship between nurses and physicians.)

The borrowed servant criteria for vicarious responsibility applies nicely to the case of decisions made by a machine in a hospital setting. The underlying approach is that an attending physician is responsible for an agent's decision to the extent that the physician has control over those decisions or the manner in which the agent (machine or human) makes its decisions. The wide range of situations and manners of control to be found in the traditional cases of a borrowed human servant will also be found in the case of borrowed machine agents. At issue is whether the clinician selects the machine from available machines, whether he or she has made a practice of supervising machine action, etc. What we need are criteria for determining when a machine judgment is within the scope of authority of the "physician in charge." It is hardly surprising that these criteria turn out to be very much like those used to determine when staff judgments are within the scope or authority of a physician. We must determine, it seems, when a machine is a borrowed servant of the doctor.

It is important to limit the doctor's accountability for machine judgment if we wish to encourage use of intelligent machines. Note that the underlying principle of the borrowed servant approach to machine judgment is that we determine whether the physician is accountable by asking whether he or she is in control. This is a formal recognition of the concern noted above that M.D.s stay in control over whatever they are held accountable for. The machines will be used only if physicians are assured that when they relinquish control to a machine, they will not continue to be held accountable.

Now let us consider M.D. use of expert systems that assist in the diagnosis of patient conditions and suggest tests or treatment. In contrast to monitoring systems that respond to patient conditions, these are usually fed information by humans and respond with suggestions. There are systems in use that make exceptionally reliable judgments (when compared to human judgment) within well-defined areas of medical concern. For instance, machines are excellent aids to determining the source of abdominal pain, often a difficult judgment (Adams et al. 1986; Waxman and Worley 1990; de Dombal, Dallos, and McAdam 1991; cf. Chapter 6). It is initially reasonable to hold a person who relies upon or rejects a machine judgment of this sort to the same level of accountability as one who relies upon or rejects the judgment of a human expert. (Averill 1984 investigates several consequences of the analogy between human experts and machine experts.) Just as physicians do not override specialists without good reason, they should not override intelligent machines without good reason. A guess or a distrust of machines is not a good reason for rejecting a machine judgment. The particular wish of a well-informed patient is a good reason. Just as doctors are expected to notice when specialists should be called in, they should notice when available machine support is called for.

Attributing duties to computers

Whether the doctor is accountable for a specialist's judgment is a question of the distribution of duties between the doctor and the specialist. Duties are widely distributed in modern medicine. We may take note of the familiar clichés (much attacked in recent literature) that M.D.s are responsible for diagnoses, pharmacists for the preparation of drugs, nurses for daily care, laboratory technicians for performing tests, etc. By treating machines as agents, some duties that traditionally belong to M.D.s (and the consequent accountability for performance of these duties) may be passed from the physician to the machine.

Among the duties that traditionally define the physician's profession are diagnosis and prescription of treatment. As noted above, one source of resistance by doctors to reliance on automated expert systems is that it feels like a partial abandonment of their distinctive role. (A doctor-basher might suggest that it also disturbs a cherished elitist attitude: Although the laborer's work may be "mechanizable," certainly the much-celebrated professional expertise of a doctor is not like that! This is unfair to a profession distinguished by its common sense.)

There are at least two possible reactions to this problem: (1) recognize that not all the duties of diagnosis belong to the physician in charge, and (2) redefine those judgments that can be automated so that they are no longer part of diagnosis. The latter approach is actually quite common. In areas where we have already accepted machine decisions, we tend not to think of the decisions as diagnostic.

We can see this transition taking place in changing physician attitudes toward electrocardiogram interpretation (Dassen, Mulleneers, den Dulk, and Talmon 1993; Rautaharju 1993; Hillson, Connelly, and Liu 1995; cf. Willems et al. 1991). Modern ECG machines provide a printout of both the data and the diagnosis. Although the ECG is often overread by attending physicians, this is no longer commonplace. We can note the change in attitude in disputes over whether ECG interpretation is billable to the patient. The U.S. Health Care Financing Administration, which administers the Medicare and Medicaid programs for elderly and low-income people, at one point decided to stop reimbursement for ECG interpretation, but reversed its decision under pressure from the medical community (see Health Care Financing Administration [no date] for a collection of reimbursement policies). Sooner or later, this decision will be reversed again – when responsibility is fully handed over to the machines. Going one step farther, "programmable pacemakers" combine diagnostic and therapeutic functions. A handheld programmer placed over certain pacemakers (sometimes known as "implanted electrophysiology labs") provides a diagnosis of the patient's changing condition.

Once the decision to react to the patient's condition is conceptually moved from diagnosis and prescription into treatment, the doctor may put the patient under control of the machine without giving up any traditional duty. In this situation we pass decisions to the machine while definitionally preserving the physician's sense of his or her traditional role. (This may explain a phenomenon reported to me by friends working in a hospital to develop expert systems for diagnostic assistance: The M.D.s were very happy to appeal to the machine's conclusions, but they viewed operation of the machines as a task for medical assistants. The machines, therefore, had to be reprogrammed, making fewer assumptions about the level of medical expertise of the operator.)

For our purposes in this chapter, it is more interesting to view the machine decision as a diagnosis, such as that made by a consulting physician. That is, the duty to make an informed diagnosis is passed to the machine. There are of course problems with the very notion of assigning duties to machines. Since machines do not enter into agreements with patients, we cannot assign them duties on a theory of contracts. In fact, I doubt that we could ever say that a machine has "accepted" a duty. But a machine might all the same have a "general duty" to whoever may be harmed by its judgment. In this sense, negligence by a pharmacist in the preparation of a drug distributed by a third party to a patient may be a tortious failure of duty by the pharmacist to the patient, even if there is no agreement between pharmacist and patient. Using this model for tracing duties through intermediaries, it is reasonable to ask whether the principal M.D. is relieved of any personal responsibility for a decision made by the consulted machine. I now suggest that, in some contexts, we may make this determination on criteria which are similar to those used when duties are assigned to humans experts.

Part of the difficulty in assigning a duty of diagnosis to a machine is that we tend to think of computerized medical decisions as performed on passive patients. The automatic defibrillator does not ask the patient if he or she wants treatment. In contrast, physicians, at least in modern medicine, are expected to explain diagnoses and treatment options to patients whenever that is reasonable (noting, of course, exceptions such as procedures performed when their urgent need is discovered during surgery intended for unrelated problems). Traditionally, computerized expert systems do not do this. In fact, they are generally bad at assessing individual patient needs. They can recommend a treatment on the grounds that 85 percent of patients with a certain profile will respond positively to the treatment. But they rarely assess the individual's biases and what the patient thinks of that form of treatment (see the point about shared decision making in Chapter 6).

If the interaction is with the attending physician and not the expert computer, then the attending physician remains accountable and cannot be said to have passed the duty of diagnosis to the machine. Once again, this reasonable approach to accountability is entirely parallel to the usual assessment of responsibility for human consultation. Accountability depends on whether the physician has passed paramount authority to the specialist and thereby abandoned some personal duties that were previously owed the patient. Although doctors frequently send patients to specialists who then take paramount authority for judgments within the scope of their specialization, the doctors who stay in attendance, interpreting the experts' advice for the patient, still have duties and are accountable for the actions of the experts. If we assign the duty of interpretation to the M.D. who interacts with the patient, we also assign that M.D. the duty to make sure the diagnosis is within professional standards, whether that diagnosis was made by human or machine.

The model of accountability offered here explains one feature of professional resistance to the use of computerized expert systems, which otherwise seems like a stubborn refusal to use machines that invade the physician's domain of diagnosis. The problem is not that the diagnosis has been given over to another, but that this has been done without passing over the *duty* of diagnosis to that other. This is a problem that may, in part, be resolved by changing the formats used by computerized expert systems. A typical system generates a range of differential diagnoses with probabilities of correctness and suggestions of tests for further determination. Physicians show greater acceptance, however, of a system that presents relevant case histories drawn from its data base. To the computer programmer, it may seem that the informational content of two presentations is more or less the same – the process that pinpoints the relevant cases is the same as the process that determine the probable diagnoses. But physicians prefer the presentation of case histories because it seems less like an imposition on the judgment process for which they will be held accountable.

I suggest that human consultants also give advice in this form during discussions with attending physicians (as opposed to consultants who meet directly with the patient). Rather than announce that the patient has measles, the consultant tells about similar cases when the patient has true measles or false measles. So the preference for expert systems that give case histories is a matter of the "right form" for expert consultations. And the right form is, in part, dictated by the level of accountability that the doctor assigns to the expert's advice. (Physicians will also point out, of course, that incidental information in the case history tends to be glossed over in a simple diagnosis.)

Justice and utility

This account avoids the questions that are traditionally asked concerning who caused a harm. There is little discussion here of how to determine whether a particular harm was within the zone of foreseeable risk for the machine error. There is no attempt to assure just compensation to all injured patients. Instead, the discussion seeks ways to encourage the use of good technology by absolving the clinician of some accountability. Rather than ask who did what, the present chapter asks how to promote certain social goods by choosing between theories of accountability. Those who object to "utilitarianism" as a coldly economic analysis of legal liability without regard to justice will find this discussion to be utilitarian in the worst way.

The utilitarian attitude of the above argument is particularly striking since it is set in the context of tort law for personal liability. That law is largely derived from a common-law tradition that looks to the notions of duty, cause, and professional judgment to determine who is truly culpable. In this chapter, however, even the notion of duty is seen as a variable to be shifted or redefined to accommodate social goods.

Indeed, I generally dislike utilitarian analyses of accountability and prefer to lay liability at the feet of those who justly deserve it. And yet the utilitarian approach seems reasonable in special contexts. There are many examples of this in medical tort law. It has been noted, for instance, that traditional liability law had a chilling effect on good Samaritans (Ratcliffe 1966). Recognizing this, many states grant an exception to liability law to encourage good Samaritanism on the grounds that it is a valuable social good (see Hattis 1989 for a review).

The present approach to responsibility in cases of dependence on machines is, if successful, an example of one more context in which a utilitarian analysis of accountability works, without committing us to this view of responsibility in general.

References

Adams, I.D., Chan, M., Clifford, P.C., Cooke, W.M., Dallos, V., de Dombal, F.T., Edwards, M.H., Hancock, D.M., Hewett, D.J., McIntyre, N., et al. 1986. Computer aided diagnosis of acute abdominal pain: a multicentre study. *British Medical Journal* 293: 800–4

Agich, G.J., ed. 1982. *Responsibility in Health Care.* Dordrecht: Reidel.

Anderson, J.G., and Jay, S.J., eds. 1987. *Use and Impact of Computers in Clinical Medicine.* New York: Springer-Verlag.

Anderson, J.G., Aydin, C.E., and Jay, S.J., eds. 1994. *Evaluating Health Care Information Systems: Methods and Applications.* Thousand Oaks, Calif.: Sage.

Averill, K.H. 1984. Computers in the courtroom: using computer diagnosis as expert opinion. *Computer Law Journal* 5: 217–31.

Bowers, S.A. 1986. Precedent-setting professional liability claims involving optometry. *Journal of the American Optometry Association* 57: 397–401.

Dassen, W.R., Mulleneers, R.G., den Dulk, K., and Talmon, J.L. 1993. Artificial neural networks and ECG interpretation: use and abuse. *Journal of Electrocardiology* 26 (Suppl. 1): 61–5.

de Dombal, F.T., Dallos, V., McAdam, W.A. 1991. Can computer aided teaching packages improve clinical care in patients with acute abdominal pain? *British Medical Journal* 302: 1495–7.

Fortess, E.E., and Kapp, M.B. 1985. Medical uncertainty, diagnostic testing, and legal liability. *Law, Medicine and Health Care* 13: 213–18.

Gotterbarn, D. 1995. The moral responsibility of software developers: three levels of professional software engineering. *Journal of Information Ethics* 4: 54–64.

Hattis, P. 1989. Physicians as Good Samaritans: are they liable? *Journal of the American Medical Association* 261: 1355, 1357, 1359.

Health Care Financing Administration (HCFA). No date. *Coverage Issues Manual.* Sect. 50–15, "Electrocardiographic Services."

Hillson, S.D., Connelly, D.P., and Liu, Y. 1995. The effects of computer-assisted electrocardiographic interpretation on physicians' diagnostic decisions. *Medical Decision Making* 15: 107–12.

Karcz, A., Holbrook, J., Burke, M.C., Doyle, M.J., Erdos, M.S., Friedman, M., Green, E.D., Iseke, R.J., Josephson, G.W., and Williams, K. 1993. Massachusetts emergency medicine closed malpractice claims: 1988–1990. *Annals of Emergency Medicine* 22: 553–9.

King, J.H. 1986. *The Law of Medical Malpractice in a Nutshell.* St. Paul, Minn.: West Publishing.

Leveson, N., and Turner, C. 1993. An investigation of the Therac-25 accidents. *Computer* 26: 18–41.

Miller, R.A., Schaffner, K.F., and Meisel, A. 1985. Ethical and legal issues related to the use of computer programs in clinical medicine. *Annals of Internal Medicine* 102: 529–36.

Mortimer, H. 1989. Computer-aided medicine: present and future issues of liability. *Computer Law Journal* 9: 177–203.

Moor, J.H. 1979. Are there decisions computers should never make? *Nature and System* 1: 217–29.

Neumann, P.G. 1995. *Computer-Related Risks.* New York: ACM Press.

Nissenbaum, H. 1996. Accountability in a computerized society. *Science and Engineering Ethics* 2: 25–42.

Ratcliffe, J.M., ed. 1966. *The Good Samaritan and the Law.* Garden City, N.Y.: Anchor.

Rautaharju, P.M. 1993. Will the electrocardiograph replace the electrocardiographer? *Journal of Electrocardiology* 26 (Suppl. 1): 58–63.

Satava, R.M. 1995. Virtual reality and telepresence for military medicine. *Computers in Biology and Medicine* 25: 229–36.

Siegler, M., Toulmin, S., Zimring, F.E., and Schaffner, K.F. eds. 1987. *Medical Innovation and Bad Outcomes: Legal, Social, and Ethical Responses.* Ann Arbor, Mich.: Health Administration Press.

Snapper, J.W. 1985. Responsibility for computer-based errors. *Metaphilosophy* 16: 289–95.

Waxman, H.S., and Worley, W.E. 1990. Computer-assisted adult medical diagnosis: subject review and evaluation of a new microcomputer-based system. *Medicine* 69 (3): 125–36.

Willems, J.L., Abreu-Lima, C., Arnaud, P., van Bemmel, J.H., Brohet, C., Degani, R., Denis, B., Gehring, J., Graham, I., van Herpen, G., et al. 1991. The diagnostic performance of computer programs for the interpretation of electrocardiograms. *New England Journal of Medicine* 325: 1767–73.

4

Evaluating medical information systems: social contexts and ethical challenges

JAMES G. ANDERSON AND CAROLYN E. AYDIN

Despite more than 30 years of development of computer-based medical information systems, the medical record remains largely paper-based. A major impediment to the implementation and use of these systems continues to be the lack of evaluation criteria and evaluation efforts. It is becoming apparent that the successful implementation and use of computer-based medical information systems depends on more than the transmission of technical details and the availability of systems. In fact, these systems have been characterized as radical innovations that challenge the internal stability of health care organizations. They have consequences that raise important social and ethical issues. This chapter provides a thorough historical and sociological context and analyzes how computer-based medical information systems affect (1) professional roles and practice patterns, (2) professional relations between individuals and groups, and (3) patients and patient care. In a point that is crucial for the development of health information systems, the authors argue that, aside from quality control, risk management, or fiscal efficiency, there is an ethical imperative for conducting system evaluations. This means that no commitment to computational advancement or sophistication is sufficient unless it includes a well-wrought mechanism for evaluating health computing systems in the contexts of their use. Failure to perform such evaluations becomes a shortcoming that is itself ethically blameworthy.

Introduction and history

Medical computing is not merely about medicine or computing. It is about the introduction of new tools into environments with established social norms and practices. The effects of computing systems in health care are subject to analysis not only of accuracy and performance but of acceptance by users, of consequences for social and professional interaction, and of the context of use. We suggest that system evaluation can illuminate social and ethical issues in medical computing, and in so doing improve patient care. That being the case, there is an ethical imperative for such evaluation.

Attempts to computerize clinical and research data began in the 1950s (Kaplan 1994; Collen 1995). Systems were developed to store information from the medical records at Tulane University Medical Center (Schenthal, Sweeney, and Nettleton 1960), the University of Missouri (Lindberg 1968), the U.S. Veterans Administration (Sturm 1965), and Massachusetts General Hospital (Baruch 1965), and from psychiatric records at the Institute of Living in Hartford (Hedlund 1978). Early progress, however, was difficult and slow (Donaldson 1974).

During the 1960s, pilot projects demonstrated the potential of computer systems for medical record keeping. With the advent of minicomputers, the 1970s saw the development of operational clinical record systems (Stead 1989). By the 1980s, computer technology permitted the development of integrated medical information systems. These systems receive patient information from multiple locations, process it, maintain clinical and financial databases, and make these data available throughout the system (Blum 1984, 1986).

Many clinical information systems had their origins in the 1960s and 1970s. The Technicon Medical Information System (Blum 1984), the HELP system (Pryor, Gardner, Clayton, and Warner 1983) and the PROMIS system (Weed 1968) represented different approaches to the automation of hospital information. During the same period, automated ambulatory medical record systems were also under development; these included COSTAR (Barnett et al. 1982), RMRS (McDonald et al. 1992), and TMR (Hammond and Stead 1986; Stead and Hammond 1988). Anderson (1992a, b) compares both types of system and reviews their acceptance and impact.

The transformation of health data

Major advances in collecting, recording, storing, and communicating medical data in the 1990s have made computer-based patient record systems feasible. Advantages of such systems include (1) improved management of and access to the medical record to improve patient care; (2) automatic review of the patient record to provide clinical decision support, control costs, and improve quality of care; and (3) analysis of clinical and financial databases to guide health care practices and policies (McDonald and Tierney 1988; McDonald 1989; Anderson 1994).

Health care reform and the growth of managed care are accelerating the implementation of information technology in health care. As a result, health care administrators are investing heavily in integrated information systems. More than half of the respondents to the Fourth Annual Leadership Survey sponsored by Hewlett-Packard and the Healthcare Information and Management Systems Society predicted that computer-based patient record systems will be ready for implementation within five years (Hewlett-Packard 1993). Much of this investment is motivated by an attempt to reduce costs. At the same time, 60 percent of the respondents to the survey ranked clinical decision support as the application that has the most potential for improving the quality of patient care.

In the United States, the Institute of Medicine (IOM) has recommended that health care professionals and organizations adopt the computer-based patient record as the standard for medical and all other records related to patient care (Dick and Steen 1991: 6). Also, one of the goals of the High Performance Computing and Communication Initiative is to provide supercomputer capability to the biomedical community. It has been estimated that widespread implementation of computer-based patient record systems in the United States could result in savings of as much as $80 billion annually (Riflking 1993).

Despite more than 30 years of development, however, the medical record remains largely paper-based. This results in major limitations in content, format, access, retrieval, and linkages of patient data. Moreover, it has been estimated that physicians spend 38 percent of their time (Mamlin and Baker 1973), and nurses 50 percent (Korpman and Lincoln 1988), in entering and retrieving information from the medical record. As much as 39 percent of hospitals' operating costs has been attributed to this type of information processing (Richart 1970).

Users, institutions, and patient care

The IOM report cites a number of ways that computer-based patient records could affect the costs and quality of patient care (Dick and Steen 1991). These include (1) improved quality of and access to clinical data; (2) integration of patient data over time and among practice settings; (3) increased accessibility of medical knowledge used by practitioners in providing care; and (4) reduction in redundant tests and services, and clerical and administrative costs. However, U.S. General Accounting Office studies (1980, 1987) of the benefits of medical information systems give limited evidence that implementation of these systems leads to cost savings. Also, few health care institutions achieve their potential benefits. One survey of 620 hospitals concluded that most hospitals use less than one-quarter of the abilities built into their computer systems (Gardner 1990).

In addition, user resistance can undermine the effectiveness of computer information systems. An early survey of 32 clinical computer applications reported in the literature over a five-year period found that more than half of the projects had been abandoned or suspended. Only 19 percent of the systems were in routine use in the hospitals surveyed (Friedman and Gustafson 1977). A later survey of 40 randomly selected hospitals found staff interference with the implementation and use of medical computer-based information systems in nearly half of the hospitals (Dowling 1980).

It is important to evaluate the limited acceptance of clinical information systems by health care practitioners. Many technological innovations in health care are diffused quickly in the medical community before their cost-effectiveness has been established (National Academy of Sciences 1979). The contrast presented by medical information systems is even more striking, since surveys indicate that physicians generally recognize the potential of computers to improve patient care (Teach and Shortliffe 1981; Singer, Sacks, Lucente, and Chalmers 1983; Anderson, Jay, Schweer, and Anderson 1986a).

It is becoming evident that the successful implementation and use of computer-based medical information systems depends on "more than the transmission of technical details and the availability of systems" (Anderson and Jay 1987a: 4). In fact, these systems have been characterized as radical innovations that challenge the internal stability of health care organizations (Zaltman, Duncan, and Holbeck 1973). They have consequences that raise important social and ethical issues (Brenner and Logan 1980; Anderson and Jay 1987c, 1990a, b; Anderson 1992c). Goodman (1994: 12–13) has observed that "science and ethics are rarely so thoroughly intertwined as in medical computing. Proper use and growth of medical computing systems must be accompanied by rigorous testing and evaluation procedures. Put differently, thorough science and engineering are necessary conditions for ethical practice."

Evaluation studies that focus on the ways these social and ethical issues interact with the implementation of clinical information systems can help predict such systems' effects on health care delivery. An earlier work brought together major research findings concerning the factors that affect the adoption, diffusion, use, and impact of computer systems in clinical medicine (Anderson and Jay 1987a). A second volume provides a guide for evaluating the effects of computerized information systems on organizational structure, work life of individuals and professional groups, and the cost-effectiveness of health care (Anderson, Aydin, and Jay 1994).

Ten questions have been useful as signposts in system evaluation (Anderson and Aydin 1994):

- Does the system work as designed?
- Is it used as anticipated?
- Does it produce the desired results?
- Does it work better than the procedures it replaced?
- Is it cost-effective?
- How well have individuals been trained to use it?
- What are the anticipated long-term effects on how departments interact?
- What are the long-term effects on the delivery of medical care?
- Will the system have an impact on control in the organization?
- To what extent do effects depend on practice setting?

In what follows here, we highlight a number of these issues by suggesting how computer-based medical information systems affect (1) professional roles and practice patterns, (2) professional relations between individuals and groups, and (3) patients and patient care. Seen properly, each of these domains illustrates the ethical importance of system evaluation (Anderson, Aydin, and Kaplan 1995).

Professional roles and practice patterns

One reason physicians have been slow to adopt medical information systems may have to do with the nature of their professional values. Freidson (1970a) describes how the training of physicians leads to a firm belief in the importance of individual judgment based on personal clinical experience. This emphasis on the primacy of clinical experience results in resistance to rules and standards based on abstract scientific findings or created by administrative or professional groups. Physicians in general are skeptical about knowledge that is outside their own experience and about attempts to standardize the practice of medicine through protocols and guidelines (Tanenbaum 1993). Medical information systems require physicians to standardize the many aspects of their practice pertaining to the recording and use of clinical information. Some systems embody protocols and guidelines which further standardize clinical practice. Still other systems incorporate reminders and alerts which might be perceived as challenging the physician's professional judgment.

Young (1984) points out that the medical record represents the physician's thought process. The style, content, and sequence of information reflects his or her individual practice style. Computerizing the record affects the clinical reasoning process. Unless there are significant advantages to physicians in using a structured computerized medical record, they will resist it.

Furthermore, physicians in increasing numbers are opting for employment with for-profit ambulatory care centers, HMOs, and other managed care organizations that offer them less autonomy than private practice. Half of all active U.S. physicians receive all or part of their income as salary (Stoline and Weiner 1988). Physicians fear that medical information systems will lead to a further loss of their autonomy (Schwartz 1970; Anderson and Jay 1987b, 1990a,b; Anderson 1992c).

Relman (1980, 1983) was among the first to point out that many of these new practice arrangements create conflicts of interest that differ markedly from those inherent in traditional fee-for-service arrangements. Under salaried and capitation reimbursement systems, physicians face ethical dilemmas in adhering to practice guidelines and organizational rules while serving as agents for their patients (Morreim 1994). Physicians' clinical decisions may be directly constrained or controlled. For example, the decision to admit a patient to the hospital may have to be approved by a third party, or an infectious disease consultant may have to approve the use of certain expensive antibiotic drugs. Another example is the use of computer systems by insurance companies to monitor the frequency and appropriateness of laboratory and radiological procedures ordered by physicians. Physicians are not reimbursed for these procedures if they fail to meet pre-established practice criteria.

Physician performance and institutional cost

Physician autonomy has traditionally been buttressed by the unavailability of information regarding physicians' performance. The limited opportunity to observe a physician's practice behavior and the high degree of specialization made control largely ineffective (Freidson and Rhea 1963; Freidson 1981). Administrators and the public had no way of determining the cost effectiveness of various procedures and services. As a result, physicians could not be held accountable for decisions that generate as much as 70 percent of all health care costs. Advances in information technology have provided new ways of integrating clinical and financial information. It is now possible to create individual practice profiles and to implement clinical protocols and practice guidelines. Computer-based information systems make it possible to monitor and regulate the clinical practice of physicians, nurses, and allied health workers (Gerbert and Hargreaves 1986; Anderson and Jay 1990a, b; Feinglass and Salmon 1990; Anderson 1992c).

Managers of health care organizations have strong incentives to use information to control the practice of medicine, in order to increase productivity and minimize costs. Comprehensive computer-based information systems are required for implementation of effective cost containment, risk management, and quality assurance programs. This process of corporate rationalization has shifted control over clinical practice from professional norms and standards enforced by physicians to organizational arrangements designed to monitor, structure, and ensure greater standardization in practice (Anderson 1992c). Computer-based information systems play a central role in this process.

Cost containment and quality control efforts have begun to rely on performance-based assessment of individual practitioners (Kassirer 1993, 1994). Thus patient data from institutional and third-party databases are merged to create a practice profile. This profile may evaluate a physician's performance on quality of care, use of services and cost, in comparison to prevailing norms or standards. The creation of practice profiles is greatly facilitated by the widespread implementation of computer-based patient records.

The use of these profiles raises important social and ethical issues. In some instances practice profiles are being used to make decisions about hiring, firing, disciplining, and paying physicians (McNeil, Pederson, and Gatsonis 1992; Welch, Miller, and Welch 1994). Private companies have begun to market practice profiles to third-party payers and employers. Often these are based on proprietary data, decision rules, and standards. Hospitals and managed care organizations use this information almost exclusively to control costs rather than to ensure quality of care (Winslow 1994).

Critics point to major flaws in databases that are created mostly from reimbursement claims. These include inaccurate data; little information about preventive services, postoperative care, and patient outcomes; and missing information on other sources of variability not directly related to the physician's clinical decisions (Brand, Quam, and Leatherman 1992; Iezzoni et al. 1992). Moreover, efforts to measure quality and outcomes are still rudimentary and will not be generally available for some time. There is the further issue of who will have access to data on individual physicians and health care organizations. Employers and third-party payers currently have access to these data, but it is not clear how much access should be made public to support assessments of the quality of individual physicians and organizations (Hillman 1991; Friedman 1992; also cf. Chapter 5 in this volume).

Computer-based medical information systems have a pervasive effect on other health care professionals as well. Total quality management and process re-engineering rely heavily upon information technology. In theory, by flattening organizational structures and providing employees with relevant information, workers can assume more responsibility for the tasks that they perform (Benjamin and Morton 1992; Clement 1994). However, to be effective, system design must be appropriate to the tasks performed by individuals and organizational units (Simborg and Gabler 1992; Esterhay 1993). Thus, evaluation studies are needed to examine the extent to which the success of computer-based medical information systems depends upon proper training and support, job design, and the organizational structure. All of these concerns indicate the need for comprehensive evaluation studies that go beyond the technical capabilities of the system to examine its interactions with and impacts on the social system into which it is being introduced (Anderson and Aydin 1994).

Professional relations

In addition to potential impact on individual roles and practice patterns, information system design may significantly influence the way individuals and professional groups interact (Anderson, Jay, Schweer, and Anderson 1986b; Anderson, Jay, Schweer, Anderson, and Kassing 1987; Anderson, Jay, Perry, and Anderson 1994). Comprehensive, integrated medical information systems affect professionals and professional groups whose goals often conflict. Several authors have characterized health care organizations as consisting of relatively autonomous, balkanized patient care delivery units. Administrators focus on cost-effectiveness while physicians, nurses, and other practitioners have different sets of priorities that include preservation of professional autonomy and control (Smith and Kaluzny 1975; Lindberg 1979a). These differences between and among groups may also hinder the acceptance and use of medical information systems and other information technology (Aydin 1994).

Major problems arise because these systems are used to standardize many aspects of medical practice and the medical record, requiring pervasive changes in the tasks performed by individuals and organizational units. Much organizational work, especially patient care, is characterized by exception handling and improvisation (Suchman 1983), which may have little to do with formal organizational structure, rules, and reporting requirements (Pfeffer 1982). In fact, the delegation of activities to different occupations is often determined by social expectations or legal obligations rather than any calculations of efficiency.

Data control and clinical outcomes

Rising demand for outcomes measures and other evidence of clinical efficacy constitutes an argument for greater attention to system evaluation. For a third of a century managers of health care organizations have been increasingly responsible for planning and coordinating the work of physicians, nurses, and allied health personnel. Many managers are physicians responsible for establishing standards by which to evaluate practice and manage clinical work. These organizational arrangements where physicians become subordinate to other physicians change relationships among members of the medical profession (Freidson 1985). Physician managers and practitioners have different perspectives. Managers are concerned with meeting the medical needs of patients within budgetary constraints while practitioners are concerned primarily with their patients' needs regardless of cost. These different perspectives create conflicts and tension within the medical profession (Scott 1982a, b).

Other professional and occupational groups may also respond to the demand for new information systems by attempting to negotiate continued control over the tasks and responsibilities required by licensing agencies and by their own professional norms (Aydin 1989). Institution-wide information systems frequently require departments to share a common database, making them dependent upon another department or professional group for data entry and the integrity of the data upon which their work depends. Thus, computer-based medical information systems may threaten a group's control over its own work processes or, conversely, improve its ability to work effectively.

In one medical center, for example, the pharmacy department accepted an order entry system that did not meet many of its specific needs (e.g., inventory control, patient billing) in return for regaining its consulting role on patient care units, a role that had been eliminated in previous budget cuts. The pharmacy department in another hospital regained control of order entry by conducting studies to show that it would be more cost-effective to have orders entered by pharmacy technicians than by nursing employees (Aydin 1994). In each of these examples, control over various patient care tasks was at issue, and the resulting implicit or explicit negotiations among professional groups were important in determining the success of the system.

Patients and patient care

The implementation of medical information systems has unforeseen effects on patients and their care. Indeed, the increased computerization of health care can expose patients to new risks and harms. Lives, well-being and quality of life at times are vulnerable to poor systems design and failure. At the same time, the ways in which medical computer systems are developed and implemented limit the accountability of any individual or organizational unit when systems malfunction and patients are harmed (Nissenbaum 1994; cf. Chapter 3).

A striking example of this problem involved the Therac-25, a computer-controlled radiation therapy machine. Massive overdoses of radiation therapy resulted in three deaths and severe burns to three other patients. An investigation revealed software errors, a faulty microswitch, confusing error messages, inadequate testing, exaggerated claims concerning the reliability of the system, and negligence on the part of hospital employees (Leveson and Turner 1993). Thus, responsibility for the malfunction was diffused among several organizations and many individuals.

A second example involved a computer-based pharmacy system (Collins, Miller, Spielman, and Wherry 1994). A small hospital hired consultants to design and implement a PC-based system designed to make dosages more accurate, decrease the time between prescription and treatment, and reduce costs. The system was implemented after it passed all tests and specifications that were included in the original contract. Within months, however, the hospital decided to return to its paper system because of potential risks to patients caused by medication errors. A problem was identified in the way the hospital staff interacted with the system – not in the software or hardware. The new system eliminated much of the oversight provided by staff in using the old paper-based system. As a result doctors, nurses and pharmacy staff all blamed someone else for entering the wrong information when medication errors occurred. Because the computer system created a common database used by all hospital personnel, it was impossible to attribute errors to any one person or department.

Moreover, the system included data-handling and user interface features from a warehouse inventory system. While the system met all of the original specifications, many of the problems involving errors, excessive time for data entry, and computer-generated advice that was unacceptable to physicians were not anticipated by the developers.

Computer-based systems shift responsibility for medical decisions in other ways as well. Computers are beginning to be used for clinical decision making, outcomes calculations, and prediction. For instance, Doyle et al. (1994) report the use of artificial neural networks to predict outcomes after liver transplantation. The authors point out that there is a large discrepancy between the demand for and the supply of organs. Given the high cost of transplantations, they suggest that computer programs like the one developed for liver transplant patients could be used to optimize the use of scarce resources such as organs. Perhaps so. But the use of computational tools seems in increasingly many contexts to provide an aura of objectivity. The question is whether such an impression is valid; this can be determined by robust attention to system evaluation.

New technologies that are largely computer-based also offer patients a bewildering amount of information concerning diagnoses and treatment options. Physicians may frequently respond to the clinical uncertainty by shifting the responsibility for medical decisions to patients. While some view this as empowering the patient, others view it as dumping information and responsibility onto the patient, who frequently is confused, frightened, and ill-prepared to make medical decisions (Rosenthal 1994).

An example involves the development of interactive video programs to provide patients with information about treatment choices for specific medical conditions such as benign prostatic hyperplasia. A patient enters personal data into a computer, which then accesses outcomes data appropriate for that patient. An interactive video program provides general information, treatment options, and probabilities of applicable outcomes. At the end of the session both the patient and the physician are given a synopsis of the information that was presented. The program is designed to assist patients in making informed choices among treatment options (Kasper, Mulley, and Wennberg 1992). Evaluation studies indicate that there are significant shifts in patient preferences after using the program. These shifts in patient preferences indicate decreases of about 50 percent in prostate surgery (Kasper and Fowler 1993). Evaluation studies are needed, however, to determine whether systems that shift decision making to the patient actually result in improved patient outcomes.

Advancing the science of system evaluation

The introduction of a computer-based medical information system into a health care organization can be viewed as a cybernetic process (Zaltman, Duncan, and Holbek 1973; Anderson, Aydin, and Kaplan 1995). While professional groups and organizational units seek to maintain a dynamic equilibrium, the widespread implementation of computer-based patient record systems has the potential to alter the social structure of the organization. Most of these organizations are relatively decentralized, with individual departments and practitioners making decisions regarding patient care. The installation of a computerized record affects the distribution of resources and power as well as interdepartmental relations (Keen 1980). Professional and occupational groups respond to change by attempting to negotiate continued control over their work and professional norms. Their response to computerized patient records is shaped by their perceptions of the usefulness of the system as well as the changes it brings to the performance of everyday jobs in the organization. Individuals and groups that benefit from the system (in terms of its support for essential tasks, and enhanced status and control) will readily adopt a computerized record system. Those whose work roles, status, and autonomy are adversely affected will resist the implementation of the system. This fact is underscored by studies that indicate that half of all computer-based information systems fail largely because of user resistance and staff interference (Lyytinen 1987; Lyytinen and Hirschheim 1987).

A major impediment to the adoption and diffusion of medical information systems continues to be the lack of evaluation criteria and evaluation efforts, a problem noted by Lindberg (1979b) and the U.S. Government's General Accounting Office (1980) nearly two decades ago. These systems affect patients, individual and organizational providers of health care, third-party payers, federal and state regulatory agencies, and society as a whole. Outcomes or benefits may be specified for any one or all of these groups. Professional values and norms, however, appear to be far more critical to the successful implementation of medical information systems than is the case with many other medical innovations (Brenner and Logan 1980). Comprehensive evaluation studies can help organizations weigh the potential benefits of a system for patient care against other changes or perceived negative impacts for specific constituencies. Organization leaders may also gain a better understanding of the social and ethical issues involved in system implementation, enabling them to work with physicians and other health care providers to adopt systems that can actually be shown to contribute to cost-effective delivery of quality patient care.

References

Anderson, J.G. 1992a. Medical Information Systems. In *Encyclopedia of Micro-computers*, ed. A. Kent and J.G. Williams, pp. 39–65. New York: Marcel Dekker.

Anderson, J.G. 1992b. Computerized medical record systems in ambulatory care. *Journal of Ambulatory Care Management* 15(3): 67–75.

Anderson, J.G. 1992c. The deprofessionalization of American medicine. In *Current Research on Occupations and Professions,* ed. G. Miller, pp. 241–56. New York: JAI Press.

Anderson, J.G. 1994. Computer-based patient records and changing physicians' practice patterns. *Topics in Health Information Management* 15(1): 10–23.

Anderson, J.G., and Aydin, C.E. 1994. Overview: theoretical perspectives and methodologies for the evaluation of health care information systems. In *Evaluating Health Care Information Systems: Methods and Applications,* ed. J.G. Anderson, C.E. Aydin, and S.J. Jay, pp. 5–29. Thousand Oaks, Calif.: Sage.

Anderson, J.G., Aydin, C.E., and Jay, S.J., eds. 1994. *Evaluating Health Care Information Systems: Methods and Applications.* Thousand Oaks, Calif.: Sage.

Anderson, J.G., Aydin, C.E., and Kaplan, B. 1995. An analytical framework for measuring the effectiveness/impacts of computer-based patient record systems. In *Proceedings of the 28th Hawaii International Conference on System Sciences,* vol. 4: *Information Systems: Collaboration Systems and Technology; Organizational Systems and Technology,* ed. J.F. Nunamakeer and R.H. Sprague, pp. 767–76. Los Alamitos, Calif.: IEEE Computer Society Press.

Anderson, J.G., and Jay, S.J., eds. 1987a. *Use and Impact of Computers in Clinical Medicine.* New York: Springer-Verlag.

Anderson, J.G., and Jay, S.J. 1987b. The diffusion of computer applications in medical settings. In *Use and Impact of Computers in Clinical Medicine,* ed. J.G. Anderson and S.J. Jay, pp. 3–7. New York: Springer-Verlag.

Anderson, J.G., and Jay, S.J. 1987c. Hospitals of the future. In *Use and Impact of Computers in Clinical Medicine,* ed. J.G. Anderson and S.J. Jay, pp. 343–50. New York: Springer-Verlag.

Anderson, J.G., and Jay, S.J. 1990a. Computers and the future practice of medicine: issues and options. *Cahiers de Sociologie et de Demographie Medicales* 30: 295–312.

Anderson, J.G., and Jay, S.J. 1990b. The social impact of computer technology on physicians. *Computers and Society* 20: 28–33.

Anderson, J.G., Jay, S.J., Perry, J., and Anderson, M.M. 1994. Modifying physician use of a hospital information system: a quasi-experimental study. In *Evaluating Health Care Information Systems: Methods and Applications,* ed. J.G. Anderson, C.E. Aydin, and S.J. Jay, pp. 276–87. Newbury Park, Calif.: Sage.

Anderson, J.G., Jay, S.J., Schweer, H.M., and Anderson, M.M. 1986a. Why doctors don't use computers: some empirical findings. *Journal of the Royal Society of Medicine* 79: 142–4.

Anderson, J.G., Jay, S.J., Schweer, H.M., and Anderson, M.M. 1986b. Physician utilization of computers in medical practice: policy implications based on a structural model. *Social Science and Medicine* 23: 259–67.

Anderson, J.G., Jay, S.J., Schweer, H.M., Anderson, M.M., and Kassing, D. 1987. Physician communication networks and the adoption and utilization of computer applications in medicine. In *Use and Impact of Computers in Clinical Medicine*, ed. J.G. Anderson and S.J. Jay, pp. 185–99. New York: Springer-Verlag.

Aydin, C.E. 1989. Occupational adaptation to computerized medical information systems. *Journal of Health and Social Behavior* 30:163–79.

Aydin, C.E. 1994. Professional agendas and computer-based patient records: negotiating for control. *Topics in Health Information Management* 15: 41–51.

Barnett, G.O., Zielstorff, R.D., Piggins, J., McLatchey, M., Morgan, M., Barnett, S., Shusman, D., Brown, K., Weidman-Dahl, F., and McDonnell, G. 1982. COSTAR: a comprehensive medical information system for ambulatory care. In *Proceedings of the Sixth Symposium on Computer Applications in Medical Care*, ed. B.I. Blum, pp. 8–18. Washington, D.C.: IEEE Computer Society Press.

Baruch, J.J. 1965. Hospital automation via computer time-sharing. In *Computers in Biomedical Research*, vol. 2, ed. R.W. Stacy and B.D. Waxman, pp. 291–312. New York: Academic Press.

Benjamin, R., and Morton, M. 1992. Reflections on effective application of information technology in organizations from the perspective of the management of the 90's program. In *Personal Computers and Intelligent Systems: Information Processing*, ed. R.H. Vogt, pp. 131–43. Amsterdam: North Holland.

Blum, B., ed. 1984. *Information Systems for Patient Care*. New York: Springer-Verlag.

Blum, B. 1986. *Clinical Information Systems*. New York: Springer-Verlag.

Brand, D.A., Quam, L., and Leatherman, S. 1992. Data needs of profiling systems. In *Physician Payment Review Commission Conference on Profiling*, no. 92–2, pp. 20–45. Washington, D.C.: Physician Payment Review Commission.

Brenner, D.J., and Logan, R.A. 1980. Some considerations in the diffusion of medical technologies: medical information systems. *Communication Yearbook 4*, pp. 609–23. Beverly Hills: Sage.

Clement, A. 1994. Computing at work: empowering action by "low-level users." *Communications of the ACM* 37: 3–63.

Collen, M.F. 1995. *A History of Medical Informatics in the United States 1950 to 1990*. Washington, D.C.: American Medical Informatics Association.

Collins, W.R., Miller, K.W., Spielman, B.J., and Wherry, P. 1994. How good is good enough? An ethical analysis of software construction and use. *Communications of the ACM* 37: 81–91.

Dick, R.S., and Steen, E.B., eds. 1991. *The Computer-Based Patient Record: An Essential Technology for Health Care*. Washington, D.C.: National Academy Press.

Donaldson, F.W. 1974. On-line computing in the medical profession. In *Computers in Medicine: Proceedings of the Second International Symposium*, ed. J. Rose, p. 18. London: John Wright & Sons.

Dowling, A.F. 1980. Do hospital staff interfere with computer systems implementation? *Health Care Management Review* 5:23–32. Reprinted in *Use and Impact of Computers in Clinical Medicine*, ed. J.G. Anderson and S.J. Jay, pp. 302–17. New York: Springer-Verlag, 1987.

Doyle, H.R., Dvorchik, I., Mitchell, S., Marino, I.R., Ebert, F.H., McMichael, J., and Fung, J.J. 1994. Predicting outcomes after liver transplantation: a connectionist approach. *Annals of Surgery* 219: 408–15.

Esterhay, R.J. 1993. The medical record: problem or solution? *M.D. Computing* 10: 78–80.

Feinglass, J., and Salmon, J.W. 1990. Corporatization of medicine: the use of medical management information systems to increase the clinical productivity of physicians. *International Journal of Health Services* 20: 233–52.

Freidson, E. 1970a. *Profession of Medicine.* New York: Dodd, Mead and Company.

Freidson, E. 1970b. *Professional Dominance.* New York: Atherton Press.

Freidson, E. 1981. Professional dominance and the ordering of health services: some consequences. In *Sociology of Health and Illness,* ed. P. Conrad and R. Kern, pp. 184–97. New York: St. Martin's Press.

Freidson, E. 1985. The reorganization of the medical profession. *Medical Care Review* 42: 11–35.

Freidson, E., and Rhea, B. 1963. Processes of control in a company of equals. *Social Problems* 11: 119–31.

Friedman, E. 1992. Public access to profiling information. In *Physician Payment Review Commission Conference on Profiling,* vol. 92–2, pp. 126–40. Washington, D.C.: Physician Payment Review Commission.

Friedman, R.B., and Gustafson, D.H. 1977. Computers in medicine: a critical review. *Computers and Biomedical Research* 10: 1–6.

Gardner, E. 1990. Information systems: computers' full capabilities go untapped. *Modern Healthcare,* May 28: 38–40.

General Accounting Office. 1980. *Computerized Hospital Medical Information Systems Need Further Evaluation to Ensure Benefits from Huge Investments.* Gaithersburg, Md.: General Accounting Office (AFMD-81-3, November 18).

General Accounting Office. 1987. *ADP Systems: Examination of Non-Federal Hospital Information Systems.* Gaithersburg, Md.: General Accounting Office (IMTEC-87-21, June 30).

Gerbert, B., and Hargreaves, W.A. 1986. Measuring physician behavior. *Medical Care* 24: 838–47.

Goodman, K.W. 1994. Ethics and system evaluation. *Physicians and Computers* 11(11):12–14.

Hammond, W.E., and Stead, W.W. 1986. The evolution of a computerized medical information system. In *Proceedings of the Tenth Annual Symposium on Computer Applications in Medical Care,* ed. H.F. Orthner, pp. 147–56. Silver Spring, Md.: IEEE Computer Society Press.

Hedlund, J.L. 1978. Computers in mental health: an historical overview and summary of current status. In *Proceedings of the Second Annual Symposium on Computer Applications in Medical Care,* ed. H.F. Orthner, pp. 168–83. Silver Spring, Md.: IEEE Computer Society Press.

Hewlett-Packard. 1993. Health care professionals speak out on information technology. *Advances for Medicine* 12: 11–15.

Hillman, A.L. 1991. Disclosing information and treating patients as customers: a review of selected issues. *HMO Practice* 5: 37–41.

Iezzoni, L.I., Foley, S.M., Daley, J., Hughes, J., Fisher, E.S., and Heeren, T. 1992. Comorbidities, complications, and coding bias: Does the number of diagnosis codes matter in predicting in-hospital mortality? *Journal of the American Medical Association.* 267: 2197–2203.

Kaplan, B. 1994. Reducing barriers to physician data entry for computer-based patient records. *Topics in Health Information Management* 15: 24–34.

Kasper, J.F., and Fowler, F.J. 1993. Responding to the challenge: a status report on shared decision-making programs. *HMO Practice* 7: 176–81.

Kasper, J.F., Mulley, A.G., and Wennberg, J.E. 1992. Developing shared decision-making programs to improve the quality of health care. *QRB Quality Review Bulletin* 18: 183–90.

Kassirer, J.P. 1993. The quality of care and the quality of measuring it. *New England Journal of Medicine* 329: 1263–65.

Kassirer, J.P. 1994. The use and abuse of practice profiles. *New England Journal of Medicine* 330: 634–36.

Keen, P.G.W. 1980. Information systems and organizational change. *Communications of the ACM* 24: 24–33.

Korpman, R.A., and Lincoln, T.L. 1988. The computer-stored medical record: for whom? *Journal of the American Medical Association* 259: 3454–6.

Leveson, N., and Turner, C. 1993. An investigation of the Therac-25 accidents. *Computer* 26: 18–41.

Lindberg, D.A.B. 1968. *The Computer and Medical Care.* Springfield, Ill.: Charles C. Thomas.

Lindberg, D.A.B. 1979a. The development and diffusion of a medical technology: medical information systems. In *Medical Technology and the Health Care System: A Study of the Diffusion of Equipment-embodied Technology,* pp. 201–39. Washington, D.C.: National Academy of Sciences.

Lindberg, D.A.B. 1979b. *The Growth of Medical Information Systems in the United States.* Lexington, Mass.: Lexington Books.

Lyytinen, K. 1987. Different perspectives on information systems: problems and solutions. *ACM Computing Surveys* 19: 5–46.

Lyytinen, K., and Hirschheim, R. 1987. Information systems failure – a survey and classification of empirical literature. *Oxford Surveys in Information Technology* 4: 257–309.

McDonald, C.J. 1989. Medical information systems of the future. *M.D. Computing* 6: 82–6.

McDonald, C.J., and Tierney, W.M. 1988. Computer-stored medical records. *Journal of the American Medical Association* 259: 3433–40.

McDonald, C.J., Tierney, W.M., Overhage, J.M., Martin, D.K., and Wilson, G.A. 1992. The Regenstrief Medical Record System: 20 years of experience in hospitals, clinics, and neighborhood health centers. *M.D. Computing* 9: 206–17.

McNeil, B.J., Pedersen, S.H., and Gatsonis, C. 1992. Current issues in profiles: potentials and limitations. In *Physician Payment Review Commission Conference on Profiling,* no. 92–2, pp. 46–70. Washington, D.C.: Physician Payment Review Commission.

Mamlin, J.J., and Baker, D.H. 1973. Combined time-motion and work sampling study in a general medicine clinic. *Medical Care* 11: 449–56.

Mason, R.O. 1986. Four ethical issues of the Information Age. *MIS Quarterly* 10: 4–12.

Morreim, E.H. 1994. Ethical issues in managed care: economic roots, economic resolutions. *Managed Care Medicine* 1(6): 39–43, 52–5.

National Academy of Sciences. 1979. *Medical Technology and the Health Care System.* Washington, D.C.: National Academy of Sciences.

Nissenbaum, H. 1994. Computing and accountability. *Communications of the ACM* 37: 73–80.

Pfeffer, J. 1982. *Organizations and Organization Theory.* Marshfield, Mass.: Pitman.

Pryor, T.A., Gardner, R.M., Clayton, P.D., and Warner, H.R. 1983. The HELP system. *Journal of Medical Systems* 7: 87–102.

Relman, A.S. 1980. The new medical-industrial complex. *New England Journal of Medicine* 303: 963–70.

Relman, A.S. 1983. The future of medical practice. *Health Affairs* 2: 5–19.

Richart, R.H. 1970. Evaluation of a medical data system. *Computers and Bio- medical Research* 3: 415–25.

Riflking, G. 1993. New momentum for electronic patient records. *New York Times,* May 2: Sec. 1, p. 8, National Edition.

Rosenthal, E. 1994. Hardest medical choices shift to patients. *New York Times,* January 27: A1, A13, National Edition.

Schenthal, J.E., Sweeney, J.W., and Nettleton, Jr., W. 1960. Clinical application of large scale electronic data processing apparatus: new concepts in clinical use of the electronic digital computer. *Journal of the American Medical As- sociation* 173: 6–11.

Schwartz, W.B. 1970. Medicine and the computer: the promise and problems of change. *New England Journal of Medicine* 283: 1257–64. Reprinted in *Use and Impact of Computers in Clinical Medicine*, ed. J.G. Anderson and S.J. Jay, pp. 321–35. New York: Springer-Verlag, 1987.

Scott, W.R. 1982a. Managing professional work: three models of control for health organizations. *Health Services Research* 17: 213–40.

Scott, W.R. 1982b. Health care organizations in the 1980s: the convergence of public and professional control systems. In *Contemporary Health Services: Social Science Perspectives*, ed. A.W. Johnson, O. Grusky, and B.H. Raven, pp. 177–95. Boston: Auburn House.

Simborg, D.W., and Gabler, J.M. 1992. Reengineering the traditional medical record: the view from industry. *M.D. Computing* 9: 198–200, 272.

Singer, J., Sacks, H.S., Lucente, F., and Chalmers, T.C. 1983. Physician atti- tudes toward applications of computer database systems. *Journal of the American Medical Association* 249: 1610–14.

Smith, D.B., and Kaluzny, A.D. 1975. *The White Labyrinth: Understanding the Organization of Health Care*. Berkeley, Calif.: McCutchan Publishing Corp.

Stead, W.W. 1989. A quarter-century of computer-based medical records. *M.D. Computing* 6: 75–81.

Stead, W.W., and Hammond, W.E. 1988. Computer-based medical records: the centerpiece of TMR. *M.D. Computing* 5: 48–62.

Stoline, A., and Weiner, J.P. 1988. *The New Medical Market Place*. Baltimore, Md.: Johns Hopkins University Press.

Sturm, H.M. 1965. *Technology and Manpower in the Health Services Industry, 1965–1975.* Washington, D.C.: Government Printing Office.

Suchman, L. 1983. Office procedures as practical action: models of work and system design. *ACM Transactions of Office Information Systems* 1: 320–28.

Tanenbaum, S.J. 1993. What physicians know. *New England Journal of Medi- cine* 329: 1268–76.

Teach, R.L., and Shortliffe, E.H. 1981. An analysis of physician attitudes re- garding computer-based clinical consultation systems. *Computers and Bio- medical Research* 14: 542–58.

Weed, L.L. 1968. Medical records that guide and teach. *New England Journal of Medicine* 278: 593–600, 652–7.

Welch, H.G., Miller, M.E., and Welch, W.P. 1994. Physician profiling: an analysis of inpatient practice patterns in Florida and Oregon. *New England Journal of Medicine* 330: 607–12.

Winslow, R. 1994. In health care, low cost beats high quality. *Wall Street Journal,* January 18: B1, B2.

Young, D.W. 1984. What makes doctors use computers? Discussion paper. *Journal of the Royal Society of Medicine* 77: 663-7. Reprinted in *Use and Impact of Computers in Clinical Medicine*, ed. J. G. Anderson and S. J. Jay, pp. 8–14. New York: Springer-Berlag, 1987.

Zaltman, G., Duncan, R., and Holbek, J. 1973. *Innovations and Organizations.* New York: John Wiley & Sons.

5

Health care information: access, confidentiality, and good practice

SHERI A. ALPERT

Privacy and confidentiality rights to nonintrusion and to enjoyment of control over personal information are so well known as to be regarded by some as obvious and beyond dispute. In unhappy fact, though, confidentiality protections are often meager and feckless because of the ease with which information is shared and the increasing number of people and institutions demanding some measure of access to that information. Health data are increasingly easy to share because of improvements in electronic storage and retrieval tools. These tools generally serve valid and valuable roles. But increased computing and networking power are changing the very idea of what constitutes a patient record, and this increases the "access dilemma" that was already a great challenge. The challenge may be put as follows: How can we maximize appropriate access to personal information (to improve patient care and public health) *and* minimize inappropriate or questionable access? Note that "personal information" includes not only electronic patient records, but also data about providers – physicians, nurses, and others – and their institutions. This chapter reviews the foundations of a right to privacy and seeks out an ethical framework for viewing privacy and confidentiality claims; identifies special issues and problems in the context of health computing and networks; considers the sometimes conflicting interests of patients, providers, and third parties; and sketches solutions to some of the computer-mediated problems of patient and provider confidentiality. What emerges is a robust account of confidentiality with the following overarching imperative: Individuals and institutions in practice, and society by enacting legislation, have a moral obligation to take steps to establish and maximize confidentiality safeguards. Technological and policy-based solutions to the access dilemma are proposed as practical approaches to an increasingly knotty ethical challenge.

Some passages of this chapter are adapted from Alpert 1993 and are reproduced by permission of and copyrighted © by The Hastings Center. I am grateful to Dr. Jerome Seidenfeld for suggesting some of the features of a comprehensive account of confidentiality in an electronic environment.

Introduction

One of the most striking trends in health care over the past quarter century is the increasing reliance on information technology. In the United States, for instance, nearly all major health care reform proposals introduced in the 1990s base a large percentage of cost savings on the use of information technology. Such technology is predicted to reduce administrative burdens and streamline the insurance and payment processes. While health care reform has underscored our increasing reliance on information technology and information systems, the trend began well before these debates, and is likely to continue at a brisk pace. Additionally, interconnections among these systems will increase, irrespective of health care system modifications.

The computerized or electronic patient record allows providers, patients, and payers to interact more efficiently, and in life-enhancing ways (Dick and Steen 1991). Some also argue that the electronic patient record can offer better security than paper records (Barrows and Clayton 1996). If handled improperly, however, the computerized record also has the potential to erode patient and provider privacy and confidentiality, to the detriment of the entire health care system. The trade-offs and tensions between the "need to know" and the right to confidentiality have been, and will continue to be, exacerbated by the use of information technology, particularly because no standard privacy- or confidentiality-enhancing methods are required of or used by those designing medical computer applications. As a report to the Secretary of the U.S. Department of Health and Human Services noted,

Historically, providers have stored medical information and filed health insurance claims on paper. The paper medium is cumbersome and expensive, two factors that led to the call for the use of EDI [electronic data interchange]. Ironically, it is this "negative" aspect of the paper medium (its cumbersome nature) that has minimized the risk of breaches of confidentiality. Although a breach could occur if someone gained access to health records or insurance claim forms, the magnitude of the breach was limited by the sheer difficulty of unobtrusively reviewing large numbers of records or claim forms.

From the provider perspective, EDI changes the environment dramatically. . . . Stringent security protocols may make it more difficult for intruders to access patient-identifiable data. If the security measures are overcome and access is attained, however, the electronic medium will potentially allow for remote and unauthorized review of unlimited health information. It will greatly increase the dimension of inadvertent and intentional breaches of confidentiality (Workgroup for Electronic Data Interchange 1992: appendix 4, 3–4).

This chapter examines privacy and confidentiality interests of patients, providers, and payers, as well as conflicts between and among them. Although these are the main players in most health care systems, there are others with a stake in health care data. They include employers, insurers (i.e., health, life, and disability insurers), companies in the medical field that could benefit financially from knowing who is making use of their products (e.g., pharmaceutical companies), and researchers. Additionally, society has a substantial stake in the quality of the overall health care delivery system – where quality is increasingly measured by computers.

The importance of privacy

Privacy is related to notions of solitude, autonomy, and individuality. Within some socially defined limits, privacy allows us the freedom to be who and what we are. By embracing privacy, we exercise discretion in deciding how much of our personhood and personality to share with others. We generally feel less vulnerable when we can decide for ourselves how much of our personal sphere others will be allowed to observe or scrutinize (Alpert 1995). The philosopher James Rachels describes privacy as being ''based on the idea that there is a close connection between our ability to control who has access to us and to information about us, and our ability to create and maintain different sorts of social relationships with different people'' (Rachels 1975: 292; cf. Culver et al. 1994).

Legal philosopher Anita Allen writes that privacy ''denotes a degree of inaccessibility of persons, of their mental states, and of information about them to the senses and surveillance devices of others'' (Allen 1988: 3). Ruth Gavison, a legal scholar, speaks of privacy in terms of our limited accessibility to others, arguing that it is related to ''the extent to which we are known to others [secrecy], the extent to which others have physical access to us [solitude], and the extent to which we are the subject of others' attention [anonymity]'' (Gavison 1984: 379). We enjoy our privacy ''because of our anonymity, because no one is interested in us. The moment someone becomes sufficiently interested, he may find it quite easy to take all that privacy away'' (ibid.). (For comprehensive reviews of legal issues in health care confidentiality and privacy see Gostin 1995 and Schwartz 1995.)

Privacy has also been described as being fundamental to respect, love, friendship, and trust; indeed, some argue, without privacy these relationships are inconceivable (Fried 1968: 477). Edward Bloustein has argued that we should regard privacy as a "dignitary tort" such that when it is violated, "the injury is to our individuality, to our dignity as individuals, and the legal remedy represents a social vindication of the human spirit thus threatened rather than a recompense for the loss suffered" (Bloustein 1984: 187–188).

Arnold Simmel likewise holds that privacy is related to solitude, secrecy, and autonomy, but contends that it also "implies a normative element: the right to exclusive control to access to private realms" (Simmel 1968: 480). The difficulty with that argument, as Gavison sees it, is the way it suggests that the important aspect of privacy is "the ability to choose it and see that the choice is respected" (Gavison 1984: 349). To her, this implies that once people have voluntarily disclosed something to one party, they can maintain control over subsequent dissemination by others – and that is generally not the case. Gavison argues that the legal system should make a strong and explicit commitment to privacy as a value.

If privacy encompasses the right that individuals have to exercise their autonomy and limit the extent to which others have access to their personal domain, then in the Information Age this concept is largely defined by how much personal information is available from sources other than the individual to whom it pertains. The less opportunity individuals have to limit access to information about them, or to limit the amount of personal information they must surrender to others (voluntarily or by coercion), the less privacy they have. This also involves determining when such information should be communicated or obtained, and which uses of it will be made by others.

Vital personal interests are at stake in the use of personal data by public and private sector organizations: "Such activities threaten personal integrity and autonomy of individuals, who traditionally have lacked control over how others use information about them in decision making. The storage of personal data can be used to limit opportunity and to encourage conformity" (Flaherty 1989: 8). The stakes here are quite high. This is clear to those who fear losing insurance benefits or jobs, or suffering social stigma, when medical, behavioral, genetic, and other information cannot be safeguarded.

It is useful to distinguish between "aesthetic" and "strategic" privacy. Aesthetic privacy means that personal information is restricted as an end in itself, that is, in instances where disclosure is inherently distressing or embarrassing. (Indeed, it might be neither: It is often quite rational to want not to divulge even mundane information.) Strategic privacy is the restriction of personal information as a means to some other end. In other words, according to the authors of this distinction, "the issue is not the experience of disclosing personal information, but the longer-term consequences of doing so" (Rule, McAdam, Stearns, and Uglow 1980: 22). Both aesthetic and strategic privacy interests are at risk in the context of personally identifiable medical and health related data.

Moral foundations of medical confidentiality

There are parallel, strong, and long-standing reasons to maintain the confidentiality of patient data. Utilitarian reasons, or those that appeal to aggregate benefit, good, or happiness (see, e.g., Mill 1957; Holmes 1995), make clear that, in the absence of some degree of confidentiality, patients will not be completely forthcoming or honest in offering the facts that physicians and nurses need for successful diagnosis and treatment. This reduces good outcomes, to the detriment of the patient and, in many cases, public health. (Contrarily, utilitarianism might also be used to justify the diminution of patient and provider privacy if doing so would contribute to a more efficient and effective health care system.) Better reasons are based on the moral philosophy of deontology or Kantianism, after the philosopher Immanuel Kant (Kant 1959). On the basis of arguments about the duty to respect persons – in part, respecting them as ends in themselves and not means to an end – we are obliged on Kantian grounds to safeguard others' personal information; and they may be seen as *entitled* to such safeguards.

If a patient cannot trust a provider or institution to keep highly sensitive and personal facts confidential, a crucial foundation in the relationship between patient and provider is undermined. This fact forms a large part of the rationale for codes of ethics in many of the provider professions.

The duty for a physician to provide confidentiality to his or her patients is traced back to the Oath of Hippocrates, which states that "Whatsoever things I see or hear concerning the life of man, in any attendance on the sick or even apart therefrom, which ought not to be noised about, I will keep silent thereon, counting such things to be professional secrets" (Annas 1989: 177). This oath limits physicians; it does not create rights for patients because it creates no obligation that patients' secrets not be revealed by others (Brannigan 1992: 194).

The American Medical Association's Code of Medical Ethics recognizes the physician's obligation to preserve patient and medical record confidentiality, "to the greatest possible degree" (American Medical Association 1996: 77). It also recognizes that there may be circumstances in which the physician's greater ethical (and possibly legal) obligation is to society (e.g., cases of patient threats of bodily harm, public health reporting, and gunshot and knife wounds).

Some argue that the standard concept of medical confidentiality is no longer valid, in part because it can no longer be guaranteed. For instance, as long ago as 1982, when medical records were not highly computerized, a physician identified at least 75 health professionals at a university hospital who had legitimate access to medical information about one of his patients (Siegler 1982). While it is true that more and more parties claim legitimate need to have access to patient information, particularly in institutional settings, it is still crucial to the quality of care that patient information be protected. A major concern for patients is that revealing sensitive information will lead to bad consequences. Vincent Brannigan and Bernd Beier contend: "It is arguable that it is not the number of persons given the information, but their relationship to the patient that determines the scope of concern; there may only be a small number of persons interested in the particular patient, but disclosure to any one of them could be devastating" (Brannigan and Beier 1991: 470). They argue that the wide circle of persons many states consider to be "legitimately interested" in a person's health, including spouses or employers, can effectively destroy any rights of privacy and confidentiality.

Patients tend to expect that their communications with physicians, nurses, and other health care providers are and will remain confidential. Because patients may presume that such communications have strong legal protection, they generally feel comfortable providing intimate details to advance their medical treatment: "Patients are not likely to disclose these details freely unless they are certain that no one else, not directly involved in their care, will learn of them" (Annas 1989: 177).

However, provider-patient privilege does not necessarily keep communications between doctors and patients confidential. In the United States, for instance, the privilege, legally recognized by some 40 states, is generally applicable only in a court of law. These laws do not apply to the many situations in which a doctor or nurse is allowed or compelled by law, regulation, or long-standing practice to reveal information about the patient to outside parties. Additionally, privilege statutes apply only in cases governed by state law. The Federal Rules of Evidence, which govern practice in federal courts, provide only a psychotherapist-patient privilege, not a general physician- or nurse-patient privilege. Therefore, the clinician-patient privilege is actually a narrowly drawn rule of evidence, not recognized at common law (as is, for example, the attorney-client privilege), and available only where it is specifically provided by statute (Hendricks, Hayden and Novik 1990: 155–6).

Computers and medical privacy

As stated at the outset, health care systems increasingly rely on information technology to manage and facilitate the flow of sensitive health information. This is the result, according to a key Institute of Medicine analysis, of several entities that want better health data to "assess the health of the public and patterns of illness and injury; identify unmet . . . health needs; document patterns of health care expenditures on inappropriate, wasteful, or potentially harmful services; identify cost-effective care providers; and provide information to improve the quality of care in hospitals, practitioners' offices, clinics, and other health care settings" (Donaldson and Lohr 1994: 1). Indeed, the very fact that computers can make the collection, dissemination, and analysis of this data relatively easy and inexpensive is, in itself, often an incentive to collect more data.

Because of marked advances in computer and telecommunications technology, data do not even need to reside in the same database to be linked. The Office of Technology Assessment has noted that "patient information will no longer be maintained, accessed, or even necessarily originate with a single institution, but will instead travel among a myriad of facilities" (OTA 1993b: 9).

Moreover, "Because of the efficiency of automated systems, violations of medical confidentiality may appear to be easier. Because of the amount of data which may be included in a comprehensive patient file, the damage to the patient whose confidentiality is violated may be proportionately greater" (Walters 1982: 201–2). Without taking great care in the design and implementation of the systems developed to capture and transmit this data, significant concerns should and will be raised about individual privacy.

Medical records usually contain a large amount of personal information, much of it quite sensitive. This information is continuous, extending from cradle to grave; it is broad, covering an extraordinary variety of detail; and, with new information technologies, it is accessible as never before. Aside from the patient's name, address, age, and next of kin, there also may be names of parents; date and place of birth; marital status; race; religion; occupation; lifestyle choices; history of military service; Social Security or other national identification number; name of insurer; complaints and diagnoses; medical, social, and family history, including genetic data; previous and current treatments; an inventory of the condition of each body system; medications taken now and in the past; use of alcohol, drugs, and tobacco; diagnostic tests administered; findings; reactions; and incidents (Gellman 1984: 258). Clearly, medical records contain information that has nonmedical uses, and access to that information could be of interest to many parties. "Traditional medical records, moreover, are only a subset of automated records containing substantial health or personal information held by educators, employers, law enforcement agencies, credit and banking entities, and government agencies" (Gostin et al. 1993: 2488). As the Workgroup for Electronic Data Interchange has noted, providers' obligation to maintain the confidentiality and integrity of information "does not change with the medium of health information transmission or storage. The provider's ability to meet an obligation to maintain confidentiality, however, can be greatly affected by use of the electronic medium to store and transmit health information" (Workgroup for Electronic Data Interchange 1992: 3).

This obligation is further complicated by the fact that more and more individuals and entities are involved in health care delivery, thereby increasing the number of people who have direct access to patient records. Additionally, "electronic storage and transmission of data enable interested parties to compile information on individuals from diverse sources, making computer based health data potentially valuable to a range of groups, including pharmaceutical companies and professional liability attorneys" (Donaldson, Lohr, and Bulger 1994: 1392).

Electronic patient information cards

Any discussion of computer technology and health data should include an evaluation of electronic cards that could store and/or control access to patient records. Three general types of card technologies are available, although other types are being developed. One card is similar to an automated teller (ATM) card or regular credit card.

Another, the optical card, uses laser technology to read and write information. The third is essentially a microcomputer and is known as a "chip card." (Chip cards have several subcategories, including "smart cards," which will be emphasized here.)

The ATM-type card is the size of a credit card, is often embossed on the front with the patient's name and health care identification number, and has a magnetic stripe across the back. The stripe stores only a minimal amount of information, including name, birth date, health insurance policy number, coverage codes, and deductibles. This card could be used, in turn, to gain access to additional insurance and medical information from databases maintained by entities other than a health care provider.

Optical cards can store large quantities of information. They may be written on only once, but may be read many times. Information can be added to these cards, but not deleted (U.S. Department of Health and Human Services 1995).

Smart cards or chip cards are plastic cards that contain one or more integrated circuit chips or employ laser technology to store information. Smart cards are the only card technology that can process as well as store information (potentially the equivalent of several hundred pages). They are typically the size of a credit card and function with a read/write device and a terminal that provides access to a host computer. The information stored on the smart card's microchip must be customized for every individual and may contain comprehensive medical and insurance information. The cards can store information about personal finances, government benefits, driving records, credit transactions, genetic predispositions, sexual orientation, immigration status, and on and on. So far, most card designs are limited to a single aspect of the cardholder's life, although this will likely change.

Through the mid-1990s, European nations embraced smart cards at a much brisker rate than the United States. For instance, approximately 80 million smart cards are being used by the German government to coordinate health benefits, and France has begun using smart cards in health administration (Seidman 1995). Data protection issues raised by smart card technologies are being explored in Europe, although, for instance, "at present, no social, political, or legal consensus has been reached about the appropriate use of the chip card in the provision of medical services in Germany" (Schwartz 1995: 327).

Smart cards can be designed to contain several "zones" which can segregate stored medical data. In one structure, there are five levels of information and access (Davies 1992: 51–3):

- Level 1: Card holder's name, gender, birthdate, next of kin, unique identification number, and possibly a personal identification number that could be used to gain access to other information on the card. All care providers could read this data, but only physicians, pharmacists, and the issuing organization could make entries.
- Level 2: Emergency information: blood type, drug allergies, prostheses,

vaccinations, etc. All care providers could read this data, but only physicians would be authorized to make entries.

- Level 3: Vaccination information: All care providers, except ambulance personnel, could access data at this level, but only physicians and nurses could make entries.
- Level 4: Medication information: prescription drugs and dosages, and allergies and intolerance to specific drugs. Only physicians and pharmacists would be allowed to read the data or make entries.
- Level 5: Medical history: all the details of a patient's medical past, including relevant information on other family members. Only physicians are permitted to read or write in this level.

Providers would be equipped with a read/write device, a computer, and software. Each provider would be given an accreditation card to gain access to data on patients' smart cards (OTA 1993b: 57). Smart cards can also encrypt data, which can authenticate both the user of the card and the integrity of the data (OTA 1993b: 58; Skolnick 1994: 188).

If medical data were completely and solely resident on smart cards it would mean that patients could have more control over that data than is afforded by any other technology. It would also mean that patients would need to be sophisticated enough to access and manipulate the storage medium and know how to segregate information on the card and how to set individual personal identification numbers to control access to sensitive information. It is likely that few patients would exercise these options, deferring instead to the care provider. Indeed, "some smart card experiments have collapsed because users have failed to understand the complex programs in the card. The many instructions and options are often ignored and are generally misunderstood. While it is true that procedures can be established to enhance security, few people use these mechanisms" (Davies 1992: 53). Additionally, it is highly unlikely that medical data will reside only on smart cards. Because of the possibility of loss of or damage to the cards, one or more backup databases will need to be created to capture data on every patient encounter.

Depending on system design, ATM-type cards might not permit patients to set access restrictions. In the absence of laws or regulations to the contrary, patients could be completely dependent on the judgment of the designers and administrators of medical and insurance databases to determine what information should be accessible to which health care provider, insurer, or other third party.

While new technology could hold the key to enhanced security procedures that restrict unauthorized access to, and disclosure of, medical and
insurance records, the technology could also allow further and broader
erosion of patient privacy. Medical data systems should be designed to
allow patients discretion in limiting access to their most sensitive health
information, particularly where there is no compelling reason to allow
access. Such control could be exercised through electronic cards, but this
would probably only affect instances of information access when the patient is present.

Patients, providers, and payers

Patient interests in confidentiality
Privacy scholar Alan Westin identified the individual's stake in the dissemination of medical data by pointing out that "the outward flow of
medical data . . . has enormous impact on people's lives. It affects decisions on whether they are hired or fired; whether they can secure business
licenses and life insurance; whether they are permitted to drive cars;
whether they are placed under police surveillance or labeled a security
risk; or even whether they can get nominated for and elected to public
office" (Westin 1976: 60).

The patient has several interests in medical confidentiality. Trust in a
physician, nurse, psychologist, or social worker is essential for effective
health care. Without trust, patients will not divulge information that may
be crucial to their care. Once trust is established, patients will generally
be open about conditions and symptoms (Annas 1989: 177).

Patients also want to ensure that sensitive information shared with a
provider remains confidential. They want their information to be released
only when they authorize the release, as to a third-party payer; they expect
that released data will be limited to information that is needed, pertinent,
and appropriate; they insist that data be disseminated only to those individuals or entities with a legitimate need for access; and they may reasonably expect that data will not be retained beyond the time required to
process and resolve claims.

In the case of biomedical research, patients *qua* subjects have an interest
in decoupling their health data from identifying information. In fact, unlinked databases (in which connections between individual identities and
health data are severed or encrypted) have often contributed to progress

in biomedicine, epidemiology, and public health while protecting confidentiality. Removal of identifying information before receipt by researchers helps provide appropriate levels of protection. Such an approach can have the effect of making some longitudinal and chart-review studies more difficult, but these difficulties can be overcome by a broad and robust commitment to valid consent for patients in research institutions, and to institutional review board scrutiny.

Use of unique identifiers. The assignment of unique identification numbers raises a variety of interesting and difficult ethical and policy issues. It is inevitable and necessary that patients be uniquely identified in a technologically sophisticated health care system. The substance of controversy in this area is in the choice of identification protocols.

In the United States, Social Security numbers (SSN) are often proposed as unique identifiers (Workgroup for Electronic Data Interchange 1992). Such use of Social Security numbers would have major policy implications, some of which would extend well beyond health care. The number is not protected by federal law from being used by the private sector for a variety of purposes, including credit, education, and insurance.

The main rationale for using the SSN is that it is already in place and would be relatively inexpensive to adopt for this new purpose. It is also generally an easy number for people to remember. A counterargument is that a number that is used in so many other aspects of individuals' lives should not also be linked to their most sensitive data.

The implication of the proliferating use of the SSN or any universal identifier is simply this: Once access to someone's SSN or identifier is gained, a floodgate of information about that individual is opened. Amassing information from various databases can result in highly detailed dossiers on individuals. Such dossiers can be used in support of adverse decisions about individuals – often in cases in which they know nothing of the decision unless or until injury is done; even then, a person may not become aware of the damage for years.

Additionally, the SSN is neither a unique number nor a reliable identifier. The U.S. Social Security Administration has estimated that some 4 million to 6 million people have more than one number (American Society for Testing and Materials 1995; Burnstein 1996); and an undetermined number of SSNs are used by more than one person, often fraudulently. The government has estimated the cost of verifying all holders of SSNs and ensuring the security and integrity of the Social Security card to be between $1.5 billion and $2 billion (U.S. House of Representatives 1991: 25).

Valid consent. The concept of informed or valid consent is a necessary component of discussions of patient privacy interests. The traditional notion is that patients, prior to authorizing the release of their medical data, know and understand the nature of the information they want released, and the party(ies) to whom it can be released. In medical treatment, "the act of consent must be voluntary, and there must be adequate disclosure of information to the patient about the data dissemination process. Patients must comprehend what they are being told about the procedure or treatment, and be competent to consent to the procedure" (OTA 1993b: 70). Successful application of the standard requirements of informed consent to the disclosure of medical information is "possible only when patients are familiar with the data contained in their records, so that they understand what they are consenting to disclose" (OTA 1993b: 70), and, presumably, to whom. Because there are inconsistent state laws providing for patients' access to their own medical records, and because patients are often not told which parts of their records are releasable, consent is in many instances not truly informed; it is therefore probably invalid.

The fact that many patients are not granted access to their own records makes them particularly vulnerable if those records are incomplete or inaccurate. By blindly consenting to a disclosure, these patients may well be putting themselves at risk in any number of ways.

Additionally, many argue that informed consent in the evolving health care system is often not voluntary. "Individuals for the most part are not [generally] in a position to forego [reimbursement] benefits, so they really have no choice whether or not to consent to disclose their medical information" (OTA 1993b: 73). Beginning in 1993, this recognition was incorporated into U.S. medical privacy legislation that would allow certain disclosures of information without an explicit consent (within fairly specific parameters, including law enforcement) (e.g., *Fair Health Information Practices Act of 1997*, 105th Cong., 1st sess., HR 52). The legislation also, however, provided for substantial penalties for disclosures that exceeded these parameters.

Independently of whether consent is granted or fully informed, only information relevant to the purpose for which it is being released should be disclosed. In other words, disclosure authorizations should not be open-ended.

Providers' interests

As more health care transactions are documented, stored, manipulated, and transmitted by computers, providers' interests will become more complex and conflicted. Such complexity and conflict emerge from ease of access to the electronic patient record – which in turn supports greater scrutiny of provider performance. Indeed, the intent of many types of outcomes research in the context of health care reform is precisely to evaluate providers' effectiveness. This is occurring in addition to other data-collection activities, most notably in the National Practitioner Data Bank. This U.S. repository contains adverse reports on practitioners, which are consolidated and sent to authorized institutions. The databank became operational in 1990; by the end of 1994 it contained more than 97,000 reports and had handled more than 4.5 million requests for information (Oshel, Croft, and Rodak 1995). Although access to the databank is restricted by federal law, pressures to contain health care costs and fraud have prompted proposals to loosen these restrictions (Wolfe 1995).

In many ways, the computerization of health records improves the quality of care: Data are accessed quickly from many locations; duplicate tests are less likely to be ordered; adverse drug interactions are more easily avoided; providers can share data more efficiently when consultations are necessary.

On the other hand, an electronic records environment may also expand a provider's responsibility and accountability to the patient because the provider is directly responsible for ensuring the accuracy of the information placed in the system, as well as for authenticating the identity of the person presenting an electronic card. If information is entered incorrectly and a patient is harmed, or if someone fraudulently uses an electronic card to receive medical care, the care provider may be held accountable.

Additionally, the lack of consistent legal protection for medical records has led to a situation in which people cannot be certain that the information they share with a provider will remain confidential. The introduction of vast computerized databases could further exacerbate this situation because providers have even less ability to ensure the confidentiality of redundantly stored patient information. As one clinician has written:

Many physicians fear progressive emasculation of the special physician-patient relationship and greater erosion of confidentiality. Our medical record threatens to become less clinically useful as we are forced to include needless . . . details while we hesitate to include important information. Likewise, physicians fear patients will become less inclined to share needed facts. . . . We are entering a critical period as physicians. Our once sacred relationship with patients is engaged to marry the technology of the Information Age. We must serve as our patients' advocates and challenge this technology to evolve in a fashion which will promote their best interests. We must oppose any attempt by third parties to use this technology to further invade the privileged and confidential information trustingly given to us by our patients. . . . We must become literate with the emerging technologies of medical information management. We cannot allow information within the medical record to further threaten patient privacy or access to health care (Oates 1992: 41).

The Office of Technology Assessment has noted that this threat to the physician-patient relationship might be used in support of denying providers, payers, researchers, and others access to information they "legitimately want and need, and that society has already deemed appropriate to give them. It could also place physicians in the difficult ethical position of deciding whether or not to enter sensitive information into the record at the patient's request (or maintaining a separate, noncomputer-based record)" (OTA 1993b: 48).

It is not difficult to conceive of a situation in which some patients and providers create a "medical underground" that operates independently of (and perhaps because of) a computerized records environment. There are many contexts in which patients do not want the fact of their medical treatment shared with others, irrespective of access controls. In some cases, patients will even incur additional expense to maximize confidentiality: Psychiatric treatment is often paid for by patients out-of-pocket, and not reimbursed through an insurance policy, precisely to avoid creating a record over which the patient has little or no control.

How serious is the problem? "I've known insurance executives who pay for their psychiatric care out of their own pockets, so that the doctor won't file a claim, and there will be no financial trail," says Dr. Jerome Biegler, a psychiatrist at the University of Chicago. "If anyone knows the problems with maintaining confidentiality, it's these guys" (Anthony 1993: 56).

Computerized medical records could exacerbate this situation by forcing patients to seek "off-the-record care" for stigmatizing conditions: maladies caused by poor hygiene; sexually transmitted diseases (from herpes to HIV); depression, stress, and substance abuse (from tobacco to heroin); and on and on. Indeed, some patients fearing bias and discrimination already ask physicians to deceive third-party payers (Dunbar and Rehm 1992). The possibility of an "off-the-record record" has even more complicating implications for physicians and nurses given the standard ethical obligation to maintain a complete and accurate chart or medical record.

Patient requests that physicians maintain incomplete treatment records could increase as confidentiality protections decrease, or become inadequate as electronic medical records evolve.

Off-the-record care also corrupts data sets used for outcomes research. Outcomes data purportedly measure the effects and effectiveness of health care, as well as patient satisfaction. To be most useful for health system analyses, standardized data elements must be captured for every patient encounter in every automated health care information system. Among standard elements is the name or identifying number of every provider and/or institution. This makes possible evaluations and comparisons of nearly every provider and health care institution, according to the Institute of Medicine (Donaldson and Lohr 1994: 71). Indeed, such evaluations and comparisons are supposed to constitute the core mechanism of managed competition (White House Domestic Policy Council 1993).

Yet such a mechanism also renders individual providers vulnerable to harm, including the loss of reputation, patients, income, employment, and, potentially, career (Donaldson and Lohr 1994:100). The more individualized the research, the greater the potential harm to a provider. This is partly due to the disaggregation of patient data, as well as lack of easy-to-cipher outcomes. Social factors are also more significant and more difficult to assess.

Public disclosure of outcome data serves an important health policy goal, but is ''only acceptable when it (i) involves information and analytic results that come from studies that have been well conducted; (ii) is based on data that can be shown to be reliable and valid for the purposes at hand, and (iii) is accompanied by appropriate educational material'' (Donaldson and Lohr 1994: 11). The Institute of Medicine also called for disclosure of data to applicable providers before public disclosure.

Third parties' interests

The rising cost of health care in Europe and North America has increased demand by payers, employers, and other third parties for data about patients and about the provider and institutions rendering care. The fundamental interest of third parties is to ensure that the care they directly or indirectly pay for is medically necessary, cost-effective, covered under their payment policies, and actually administered.

Consider the example of a business beginning the process of computerizing its employees' medical records, ostensibly to improve the efficiency of its health insurance operation. A self-insuring company, it issued a release form to each of about 9,000 employees:

> To all physicians, surgeons and other medical practitioners, all hospitals, clinics and other health care delivery facilities, all insurance carriers, insurance data service organizations and health maintenance organizations, all pension and welfare fund administrators, my current employer, all of my former employers and all other persons, agencies or entities who may have records or evidence relating to my physical or mental condition:
>
> I hereby authorize release and delivery of any and all information, records and documents (confidential or otherwise) with respect to my health and health history that you, or any of you, now have or hereafter obtain to the administrator of any employee benefit plan sponsored by Strawbridge & Clothier, any provider of health care benefits offered or financed through a benefit plan sponsored by Strawbridge & Clothier, and any insurance company providing coverage through any benefit plan sponsored by Strawbridge & Clothier (Dahir 1993: 11).

Not surprisingly, some of the employees were uncomfortable with the sweeping nature of the release authorization. Only about a dozen employees, however, challenged the form's use and, fearing that the information might be used to make employment decisions, persuaded the company to add a clause to their forms specifying that the records could be used by the insurance companies, but exclusively in processing medical claims. The company also agreed that in subsequent years, the authorization forms would be amended in the same way for the remaining 9,000 employees.

A comprehensive University of Illinois survey of employer information handling practices showed that 50 percent of the companies surveyed use employee medical records in making employment decisions. Of these, 19 percent do not inform employees of such use (Linowes 1989: 50). A 1991 Office of Technology Assessment study found that many companies will not hire people with a pre-existing medical condition (OTA 1991: 3–4), a practice that continues despite prohibitions by the Americans with Disabilities Act. This practice will become more worrisome as patient records contain additional and new kinds of information, including genetic data (Powers 1994).

Consider further that information on nearly half of the 1.6 billion prescriptions filled each year in the United States is passed along to data collectors who, in turn, sell the information to pharmaceutical companies (Miller 1992). Since the early 1990s, four of the world's largest pharmaceutical companies have purchased either discount pharmacy chains or prescription benefits managers (firms that manage administrative aspects of prescription drug benefits for insurers). At least two of the four pharmaceutical concerns have made no secret of their use of prescription information (including patient and/or provider identifiers) to promote its pharmaceutical products (Wall Street Journal 1995) or study drug effectiveness (Kolata 1994).

Additionally, many companies offer discounted computing services, including health insurance claims processing, office management, and patient tracking and billing, in exchange for other considerations. In the case of one company, part of the quid pro quo is that physicians must keep all patient records on the computer network, allowing the company to obtain aggregate clinical data for commercial and marketing purposes. The database available to this company includes "clinical data, such as age, sex, diagnosis, treatment, procedures and prescription information" (Physician Computer Network 1993: 1). Typically, these exchanges of patient information take place without patients' knowledge or consent.

Another type of access to medical records occurs through the Medical Information Bureau (MIB), a nonprofit association formed to exchange members' underwriting information as an alert against insurance fraud. With a membership of more than 600 insurance companies, its members "include virtually every major company issuing individual life, health and disability insurance in the United States and Canada" (MIB 1990: 5). According to its brochure, "MIB's basic purpose was (and continues to be) to make it much more difficult to omit or conceal significant information" (MIB 1991: 2–3). The association enters approximately 3 million coded records a year using 210 medical categories, and has information on about 15 million Americans (OTA 1993b: 32).

MIB acquires data when someone applies for medically underwritten life, health, or disability insurance from a member company (OTA 1993b: 32). If the applicant has a "condition significant to health or longevity," then member companies are required to send a brief coded report to MIB. The reports, whose accuracy is not verified by MIB, also include applicants' adverse driving records, participation in hazardous sports, and aviation activities.

Information has always been the lifeblood of business and industry. Those who control or influence the flow of information tend to thrive. This is no less true in the health professions and businesses. For our purposes the challenge, given third-party interests in health information, is this: Can organizations, including many of the companies described above, do legitimate business and at the same time not violate individual patient privacy and confidentiality? Indeed, the selling and brokering of patient and provider data are arguably inappropriate under any circumstances. The challenge is all the greater considering the somewhat reckless nature of the electronic patient record and health information universe:

> In fact, the medical records environment is so open-ended now that the American Medical Records Association has identified twelve categories of information seekers outside of the health care establishment who regularly peek at patient files for their own purposes, among them employers, government agencies, credit bureaus, insurers, education institutions, and the media. Tack onto this list unauthorized data gatherers such as private investigators and people with a vested interest in uncovering all they can about someone they want to turn a dirty deal on, and it's clear the amount of medical information making the rounds these days is monumental (Rothfeder 1992: 180).

Potential solutions

After studying the potential effects of computerizing medical information on privacy and confidentiality, the Office of Technology Assessment concluded that

> All health care information systems, whether paper or computer, present confidentiality and privacy problems. . . . Computerization can reduce some concerns about privacy in patient data and worsen others, but it also raises new problems. Computerization increases the quantity and availability of data and enhances the ability to link the data, raising concerns about new demands for information beyond those for which it was originally collected. The potential for abuse of privacy by trusted insiders to a system is of particular concern (OTA 1993a: 3; cf. OTA 1993b).

Patient information technologies offer many benefits, notably the prospect of lowering administrative costs associated with health care delivery and improving ease of access to important data by appropriate individuals. However, the existence – indeed, prevalence – of databases capturing and storing medical and insurance information means that, without special measures, patients are unlikely to control or effectively limit access to their medical records. For this reason, and the overwhelming consequences for public health, there must be legal recognition of patients' interest in privacy, and in confidentiality of medical records. The safeguards must transcend state, province, county, or region. While such protections are critical now, they will become even more important as the electronic patient record and other information storage and retrieval technologies evolve. Safeguards may be established through policy and technological applications (cf. Gaunt and Roger-France 1996).

Public policy approaches

Most European countries have omnibus data-protection laws and/or explicit constitutional provisions protecting individual privacy. These protections include medical records. Moreover, other conventions and treaties provide additional protections within Europe, including directives promulgated by the Commission of the European Union and the Council of Europe (Schwartz 1995). In some cases, however, these protections are insufficient: In Great Britain, National Health Service patient records have been obtainable, for a price, from detective agencies advertising in the telephone book (Rogers and Leppard 1995). U.S. health records are a commodity (Kolata 1995) that enjoys few national legal protections and inconsistent state protections. In the increasingly computerized environment for collecting, maintaining, using, storing, and disclosing medical records, the need for legal protections has become critical.

These protections should clearly define (1) the content of the medical record, (2) patients' rights with respect to their own medical information, (3) what constitutes legitimate access to and use of personal health and medical information, and (4) prohibited uses. Also needed are oversight and enforcement mechanisms to ensure compliance, including civil remedies and criminal penalties for prohibited activities. Legal protections should also set schedules for how long medical records may be maintained, and by whom (physicians, hospitals, insurers, etc.).

Patients should have the right to be notified of the use to which health information is put, and should be able to obtain and correct their own records. Patients should also be informed, no later than the time of data collection, of any opportunity to refuse to consent to the disclosure of their medical records, or to withdraw consent later, and the consequences of both actions. Patients should have the prerogative of limiting authorization for use and disclosure of their health information, and they should be told which records are subject to the authorization, the parties allowed access, and the expiration date for the authorization, and that they can revoke the authorization. Patient data should be obtained directly from the patient, unless he or she is unable to provide it. Mechanisms should also be put in place to audit use of patient records, to track requests for and disclosures of information, including the reasons why the information was requested. Moreover, this tracking information should be available to the patient.

Any use of unique identifiers must be prohibited for all purposes not directly related to providing health care. (For instance, in 1991, the Province of Ontario passed a law to prohibit the use of a person's health number for purposes unrelated to health administration, planning, health research, or epidemiological studies [Province of Ontario 1991].) Employers' ability to review employee medical records and use medical or health information to make employment-related decisions should be strictly limited or even prohibited, as should the marketing of personal health or medical data.

A major U.S. health insurance reform enacted in 1996 requires the establishment of networked information systems for patient and other clinical data. Unfortunately, the law addresses none of the privacy protection measures identified here. Instead, the Congress postponed these critical policy decisions for as long as four years. During this time the executive branch must adopt data-transmission standards; only thereafter must privacy and security standards be adopted.

Finally, any system of safeguards must include genetic information as a special case, worthy of additional protections. Because the most egregious wrongs that might come from inappropriate use of genetic data include the denial of health care, or of reimbursement for it, and employment and other bias, it is clear that nothing less than a national health plan and strict antidiscrimination measures can adequately protect people from the worst sort of bias wrought by failure of confidentiality protections.

Technological approaches

Data protection policies if they are to be effective in this rapidly changing environment, must not be tied to specific systems and system capabilities but, rather, must establish security protection guidelines that define system goals but do not specify how these goals will be reached. These protections will be most effective if privacy is addressed directly at the outset in developing electronic systems (Gostin et al. 1993: 2491).

From a technical standpoint, it is important to point out that no system can be made completely secure. Effective security methods can minimize vulnerability, but such protections cannot be specified in legislation because systems vary widely in structure and design, making it unrealistic to require explicit procedures and policies. (See Barber, Treacher, and Louwerse 1996 for treatments of a number of security issues.)

Brannigan stresses the fact that there are competing interests involved in the design and implementation of clinical information systems: Patients want to ensure that no one has unnecessary access to their data; hospital administrators see privacy as an impediment to getting access to data needed for management; physicians view it as a time-consuming limitation on medical practice; and information system developers find it expensive, inelegant, and time-consuming (Brannigan 1992). He warns, however, that the balance between privacy and access is not a medical or technical question, but a political one. Because patients are not well represented in the design, development, and operation of information systems, the political process must ensure that their interests are protected in these activities (Brannigan 1992). A U.S. National Research Council report, documenting the health care industry's increasing reliance on electronic medical records, warns that many of the component systems are vulnerable to abuse. The report found that there are few incentives within industry to provide comprehensive security measures to protect records, but that the need to protect them will increase as organizations more frequently rely on electronic media to store and share health data. The report makes several technological and organizational recommendations to increase the security and confidentiality of electronic health information. Technologically, the Council recommends authenticating users, controlling system access, creating audit trails, and other measures. At the organizational level, health care organizations should create security and confidentiality policies and committees, establish programs for education and training, and adopt measures that include strict sanctions for policy violations (National Research Council 1997).

Many types of standards are relevant for automated information systems. These include establishing a standard data set to define all elements to be collected during patient encounters. Data-collection standards will facilitate the exchange, matching, and aggregation of patient data from disparate places. Security standards are needed to set technical and procedural authorization limitations on access to and aggregation of patient records (American Medical Association 1996). Concomitant public policies that limit the amount and type of patient data collected are also needed.

Data-exchange standards deal with the electronic transmission of the information. Security standards can be developed to specify the use of encryption, digital signatures, and personal identification/user verification systems, including biometric safeguards (voice prints, fingerprints, and so forth) or password authentication. These types of security standards are also relevant for access to information systems.

A smart card system for maintaining medical records could provide the most secure means of providing protection, but only if the records are maintained solely on the cards. From a practical standpoint, however, and for reasons already discussed, this might not be feasible.

Probably the greatest potential threat to personal privacy in health records (paper or electronic) is from inappropriate access to information by persons authorized to use the system (OTA 1993b: 12). This is known as the threat of the "trusted insider," and it presents a difficult challenge. Fine-grained audit trails and stringent access controls, particularly in automated systems, are crucial means of protecting medical information. Access controls within an information system include user profiles which specify what data the person may see and/or modify, and they provide user-specific menus to ensure that users see only that data for which they have a specific need; such controls also define permitted actions (access, read, write, modify), combinations of actions, and durations. The Council of Europe's Draft Recommendation on the Protection of Medical Data states that member countries should take security measures to "ensure in particular the confidentiality, integrity and accuracy of processed data, as well as the protection of patients . . ." (Council of Europe 1996: 9). These measures are intended to prevent unauthorized visits to data-processing installations; keep data from being read, copied, modified, or removed by unauthorized persons; prevent unauthorized data entry, modification, or deletion; prevent unauthorized transmission of data; enable separation of identifiers, administrative data, medical data, social data, and genetic data; ensure the eligibility of the intended recipient to receive transmitted data; ensure that means are established to check who has had access to a system and/or has changed data, and when; secure the transmission of data; and make back-up copies of data to ensure availability. The Council also incorporates into the Draft Recommendation the appointment of an independent person who is responsible for information system security and data protection.

Education and training are also important elements in the protection of personal health data, both for patients and for those in the health care industry, including system designers and users (whether providers, insurers, or researchers). Patients must be made aware of the contents, dissemination, and disclosure of their medical records, so they can understand their rights. Those involved in the design and development of these systems must be sensitive to the need for accommodating privacy and confidentiality protections into their systems. Indeed, designers and users must consider patient privacy and confidentiality as critical to computer systems as treatment information and the tracking of prescriptions. Users must view these protections as a critical factor in the operation of these systems – just as critical as the systems' other components, including those that provide care to patients. System users must understand what their personal and institutional responsibilities are, both legally and ethically. Most fundamentally, however, policy makers must explicitly embrace privacy and confidentiality as goods assigned the highest ethical priority in the political arenas of the world's democracies.

With the sort of national legal rights outlined in this chapter, patients can be more confident that their health information will be covered by stringent protections that respect their dignity and their privacy. Such protections will also enhance the effectiveness of the technical and administrative security measures built into the electronic records environment of the future, and help guarantee that existing paper medical records are protected as well.

While the new information technologies pose threats to the confidentiality of our most intimate health information, forward-looking public policy can assure that the enormous power of these technologies is made to serve patients' interests, not confound them.

References

Allen, A. 1988. *Uneasy Access: Privacy for Women in a Free Society*. Totowa, N.J.: Rowman & Littlefield.

Alpert, S. 1993. Smart cards, smarter policy: medical records, privacy, and health care reform. *Hastings Center Report* 23(6): 13–23.

Alpert, S. 1995. Privacy and intelligent highways: finding the right of way. *Santa Clara Computer & High Technology Law Journal*, 11(1): 97–118.

American Medical Association. 1996. *Code of Medical Ethics: Current Opinions with Annotations*. Chicago: American Medical Association (Council on Ethical and Judicial Affairs).

American Society for Testing and Materials. 1995. *Standard Guide for Properties of a Universal Healthcare Identifier (UHID)*. W. Conshohocken, Pa.: American Society for Testing and Materials (Standard no. 1714).

Annas, G.J. 1989. *The Rights of Patients: The Basic ACLU Guide to Patient Rights*, 2nd ed. Carbondale, Ill.: Southern Illinois University Press.

Anthony, J. 1993. Who's reading your medical records? *American Health*, November: 54–7.

Barber, B., Treacher, A., and Louwerse, C.P., eds. 1996. *Towards Security in Medical Telematics: Legal and Technical Aspects*. Amsterdam: IOS Press.

Barrows, R., and Clayton, P. 1996. Privacy, confidentiality and electronic medical records. *Journal of the American Medical Informatics Association* 3: 139–48.

Bloustein, E. 1984. Privacy as an aspect of human dignity: an answer to Dean Prosser. In *Philosophical Dimensions of Privacy: An Anthology*, ed. F.D. Schoeman, pp. 156–202. Cambridge: Cambridge University Press.

Brannigan, V.M. 1992. Protecting the privacy of patient information in clinical networks: regulatory effectiveness analysis. In *Extended Clinical Consulting by Hospital Computer Networks*, Annals of the New York Academy of Sciences, vol. 670, ed. D.F. Parsons, C.N. Fleischer, and R.A. Greenes, pp. 190–201. New York: New York Academy of Sciences.

Brannigan, V.M., Beier, B. 1991. Standards for privacy in medical information systems: a technico-legal revolution. *Datenschutz und Datensicherung* 9: 467–72.

Burnstein, K. Program Specialist for Enumeration, U.S. Social Security Administration, Baltimore, personal communication, March 1996.

Council of Europe. 1996. Draft Recommendation No. R (96) of the Committee of Ministers to Member States on the Protection of Medical Data [and other Genetic Data] (and Explanatory Memorandum revised in light of decisions taken at the 30th meeting of the CJ-PD) (21–24 November 1995). Strasbourg: Council of Europe.

Culver, C., Moor, J., Duerfeldt, W., Kapp, M., and Sullivan, M. 1994. Privacy. *Professional Ethics* 3: 3–25.

Dahir, M. 1993. Your health, your privacy, your boss, *Philadelphia City Paper,* May 28–June 4: 10–11.

Davies, S. 1992. *Big Brother: Australia's Growing Web of Surveillance.* East Rosewell, N.S.W.: Simon and Schuster.

Dick, R.S., and Steen, E.B., eds. 1991. *The Computer-Based Patient Record: An Essential Technology for Health Care.* Washington, D.C.: National Academy Press (Institute of Medicine).

Donaldson, M.S., and Lohr, K.N., eds. 1994. *Health Data in the Information Age: Use, Disclosure, and Privacy.* Washington, D.C.: National Academy Press (Institute of Medicine).

Donaldson, M.S., Lohr, K.N., and Bulger, R.J. 1994. From the Institute of Medicine: Health data in the information age: use, disclosure, and privacy – part II. *Journal of the American Medical Association* 271: 1392.

Dunbar, S., and Rehm, S. 1992. On visibility: AIDS, deception by patients, and the responsibility of the doctor. *Journal of Medical Ethics* 18: 180–5.

Flaherty, D.H. 1989. *Protecting Privacy in Surveillance Societies: The Federal Republic of Germany, Sweden, France, Canada, and the United States.* Chapel Hill: University of North Carolina Press.

Fried, C. 1968. Privacy (a moral analysis). *Yale Law Journal* 77: 475–93.

Gaunt, N., and Roger-France, F. 1996. Security of the electronic health care record – professional and ethical implications. In *Towards Security in Medical Telematics: Legal and Technical Aspects,* ed. B. Barber, A. Treacher, and C.P. Louwerse, pp. 10–22. Amsterdam: IOS Press.

Gavison, R. 1984. Privacy and the limits of the law. In *Philosophical Dimensions of Privacy: An Anthology,* ed. F.D. Schoeman, pp. 346–402. Cambridge: Cambridge University Press,

Gellman, R.M. 1984. Prescribing privacy: The uncertain role of the physician in the protection of patient privacy. *North Carolina Law Review* 62: 255–94.

Gostin, L.O., Turek-Brezina, J., Powers, M., Kozloff, R., Faden, R., and Steinauer, D. 1993. Privacy and security of personal information in a new health care system. *Journal of the American Medical Association* 270: 2487–93.

Gostin, L.O. 1995. Health information privacy. *Cornell Law Review* 80: 101–84.

Hendricks, E., Hayden, T., and Novik, J.D. 1990. *Your Right to Privacy: A Ba-*

sic Guide to Legal Rights in an Information Society, 2nd ed. Carbondale,
    Ill.: Southern Illinois University Press (American Civil Liberties Union).
Holmes, R. 1995. Privacy: Philosophical foundations and moral dilemmas. In
    Privacy Disputed, ed. P. Ippel, G. de Heij, and B. Crouwers, pp. 15–29.
    The Hague: SDU.
Kant, I. 1959. *Foundations of the Metaphysics of Morals.* Translated by L.W.
    Beck. Indianapolis: Bobbs-Merrill. (The *Grundlegung zur Metaphysik der
    Sitten* was originally published in 1785.)
Kolata, G. 1994. New frontier in research: mining patient records. *New York
    Times,* August 9: A11, National Edition.
Kolata, G. 1995. When patients' records are commodities for sale. *New York
    Times,* November 15: A1, B7, National Edition.
Linowes, D.F. 1989. *Privacy in America: Is Your Private Life in the Public
    Eye?* Urbana, Ill.: University of Illinois Press.
Medical Information Bureau (MIB). 1991. *The Consumer's MIB Fact Sheet.*
    Westwood, Mass.: Medical Information Bureau.
Medical Information Bureau (MIB). 1990. *MIB, Inc.: A Consumer's Guide.*
    Westwood, Mass.: Medical Information Bureau.
Mill, J.S. 1957. *Utilitarianism.* Indianapolis: Bobbs-Merrill. (Originally pub-
    lished in 1861.)
Miller, M.W. 1992. Patients' records are treasure trove for budding industry.
    Wall Street Journal, February 27: A1, A6, East Coast Edition.
National Research Council. 1997. *For the Record: Protecting Electronic Health
    Information.* Washington, D.C.: National Academy Press.
Oates, R. 1992. Confidentiality and privacy from the physician perspective. In
    the *Compendium of the First Annual Confidentiality Symposium of the
    American Health Information Management Association,* Washington, D.C.,
    July 15, pp. 138–43.
Office of Technology Assessment (OTA). 1991. *Medical Monitoring and
    Screening in the Workplace: Results of a Survey – Background Paper.*
    Washington, D.C.: U.S. Government Printing Office (OTA-BP-BA-67).
Office of Technology Assessment (OTA). 1993a. *Report Brief: Protecting Pri-
    vacy in Computerized Medical Information.* Washington, D.C.: U.S.
    Government Printing Office.
Office of Technology Assessment (OTA). 1993b. *Protecting Privacy in Comput-
    erized Medical Information.* Washington, D.C.: U.S. Government Printing
    Office (OTA-TCT-576).
Oshel, R.E., Croft, T., and Rodak, J. 1995. The National Practitioner Data Bank:
    the first 4 years. *Public Health Reports* 110: 383–94.
Physician Computer Network, Inc. 1993. *Annual Report for 1992.* Lawrence
    Harbor, N.J.
Powers, M. 1994. Privacy and the control of genetic information. In *The Ge-
    netic Frontier: Ethics, Law, and Policy,* ed. M.S. Frankel and A. Teich, pp.
    77–100. Washington, D.C.: American Association for the Advancement of
    Science.
Province of Ontario 1991. Health Cards and Numbers Control Act. Statutes of
    Ontario 1991, Chapter 1.
Rachels, J. 1975. Why is privacy important? *Philosophy & Public Affairs* 4(4):
    323–33. Reprinted in *Philosophical Dimensions of Privacy: An Anthology,*
    ed. F.D. Schoeman, pp. 290–299, Cambridge: Cambridge University Press,
    1984.

Rogers, L., and Leppard, D. 1995. For sale: Your secret medical records for £150. *Sunday Times*, London, November 26: 1.

Rothfeder, J. 1992. *Privacy for Sale*. New York: Simon & Schuster.

Rule, J., McAdam, D., Stearns, L., and Uglow, D. 1980. *The Politics of Privacy*. New York: New American Library.

Schwartz, P. 1995. The protection of privacy in health care reform. *Vanderbilt Law Review* 48: 295–347.

Seidman, S. 1995. Introduction to smart card technology and applications. In *CardTech/SecurTech '95 Conference Proceedings,* pp. 1–16. Rockville, Md.: CardTech/SecurTech.

Siegler, M. 1982. Confidentiality in medicine – a decrepit concept. *New England Journal of Medicine* 307: 1518–21.

Simmel, A. 1968. *International Encyclopedia of the Social Sciences,* s.v. "privacy."

Skolnick, A.A. 1994. Protecting privacy of computerized patient information may lie in the cards. *Journal of the American Medical Association* 272: 187–9.

U.S. Department of Health and Human Services. 1995. Final report of the Task Force on the Privacy of Private-Sector Health Records. (Kunitz and Associates, Inc., under Department of Health and Human Services Contract HHS-100–91–0036.) Rockville, Md.: U.S. Department of Health and Human Services.

U.S. House of Representatives. 1991. *Use of Social Security Number as a National Identifier.* Subcommittee on Social Security of the Committee on Ways and Means, 102nd Cong., 1st sess., February 27, Serial 102–11 (Gwendolyn King, Commissioner of the U.S. Social Security Administration, speaking on integrity of Social Security numbers).

Wall Street Journal. 1995. Eli Lilly plans to use PCS unit's database to boost drug sales. *Wall Street Journal,* May 11: B6, West Coast Edition.

Walters, L. 1982. Ethical aspects of medical confidentiality. In *Contemporary Issues in Bioethics*, 2nd ed., eds. T.L. Beauchamp and L. Walters, pp. 198–203. Belmont, Calif.: Wadsworth. First published in *Journal of Clinical Computing* 4 (1974): 9–20.

Westin, A.F. 1976. *Computers, Health Records, and Citizen's Rights.* Washington, D.C.: United States Department of Commerce.

White House Domestic Policy Council. 1993. *The President's Health Security Plan.* New York: Times Books.

Wolfe, S.M. 1995. Congress should open the National Practitioner Data Bank to all. *Public Health Reports* 110: 378–9.

Workgroup for Electronic Data Interchange. 1992. *Report to the Secretary of the U.S. Department of Health and Human Services.* Washington, D.C.: Workgroup for Electronic Data Interchange.

6

Ethical challenges in the use of decision-support software in clinical practice

RANDOLPH A. MILLER AND
KENNETH W. GOODMAN

Sophisticated machines to assist human cognition, including decision making, are among the most interesting, important, and controversial machines in the history of civilization. Debates over the foundations, limits, and significance of artificial intelligence, for instance, are exciting because of what we learn about being human, and about what being human is good for. Decision-support systems in the health professions pose similarly exciting challenges for clinicians, patients, and society. If humans have had to accept the fact that machines drill better holes, paint straighter lines, have better memory ... well, that is just the way the world is. But to suggest that machines can think better or more efficiently or to greater effect is to issue an extraordinary challenge. If it were clear that this were the case – that computers could replicate or improve the finest or most excellent human decisions – then claims to functional uniqueness would need to be revised or abandoned. Clinical decision making enjoys or tries to enjoy status at the apex of rational human cognition, in part because of the richness of human biology and its enemies, and in part because of the stakes involved: An error at chess or chessboard manufacture is disappointing or costly or vexing, but generally not painful, disabling, or fatal. This chapter explores the loci of key ethical issues that arise when decision-support systems are used, or their use is contemplated, in health care. These issues are of appropriate use and users, of the relationship to clinical care standards, and of traditional professional-patient relationships. The authors argue that these issues are best addressed by attention to traditional understanding of appropriate tool use, and to a robust intention to proceed cautiously – a position further developed in Chapters 7 and 8, on the use of prognostic scoring systems and meta-analysis.

Introduction

Medical decision-support systems (MDSS) are computer programs that help health care professionals make decisions regarding patient care (Shortliffe 1987). Use of simple or even primitive decision-support sys-

102

tems is ubiquitous, and the degree of sophistication of the MDSS in general use has increased over time (Miller 1994). Medical computing applications have a broad, indeed a vast, range of abilities. They help physicians and nurses to calculate drug dosages, warn prescribers and pharmacists of possible drug interactions, assist ICU personnel in calculating intravenous fluid drip rates, assist physicians and respiratory therapists in the interpretation of arterial blood gas results, help clinicians to read electrocardiograms and to monitor hospitalized patients for arrhythmias, and aid clinicians in locating relevant references from the medical literature. Some programs can already suggest diagnoses or therapies, and it is likely that such programs, as they improve, will be used more heavily in the future. The expansion of managed competition, especially in North America, is also likely to increase the use and importance of MDSS and other types of clinical computer programs, devices, and tools, including electronic medical records.

Because decision-support systems affect patients' health and well-being, ethical issues arise regarding their use; this was first seen more than a decade ago (Miller, Schaffner, and Meisel 1985). The most important ethical issues that arise in the use of clinical decision-support systems are these:

- Why and when should an MDSS be used?
- How should a given system be used, in what contexts, and by whom?
- What is and what should be the influence of decision-support systems on the standard of medical care?
- Will such systems alter the traditional physician- or professional-patient relationship?

This chapter expands on these questions, and suggests answers to them.

Why and when to use an MDSS

Medical decision-support systems should be used for the same reason that any standard medical device or tool is used: to improve health care outcomes and the process of health care delivery. The ultimate measure of both is improved patient well-being. Such well-being applies to the community of patients served by the health care practitioner, as well as to individual patients. It is clear that busy practitioners make compromises between learning everything that might be relevant to delivering optimal care to each patient and delivering care efficiently and effectively to a large number of patients (Covell, Uman, and Manning 1985; Osheroff et al. 1991). One might spend weeks in a medical library and in consultation with experts before deciding the precise, optimal therapy for each patient. Such an approach is impractical and harmful to those patients who would not receive care from the practitioner sequestered in a library. Moreover, for many caregivers in ordinary practice, using an MDSS to generate diagnoses for every patient would be like giving motorcycles to monks: The technology might just not be relevant in the majority of cases. Thus, the pragmatic question of when to use an MDSS is not easy to answer.

Medical decision-support systems are in most respects no different from any other tool commonly used in clinical practice. Tools like the stethoscope extend the native abilities of the clinician. Yet, just as the stethoscope augments hearing but does not replace what goes on between the ears, tools for decision-support cannot and should not replace the clinician (Miller 1990). MDSSs should be used when the health care practitioner encounters a question or problem that may be efficiently and effectively answered through the use of the system.

The mere availability of an MDSS does not provide adequate justification for its use on all patients in all situations. The properly trained clinician knows how and when to use a stethoscope, although the level of skill varies between, say, cardiologists and other health care professionals. It is not necessary to examine the heart and lungs of a healthy 18-year-old male who earlier had a normal exam and who presents to the clinic for suturing of a minor laceration sustained while playing football. Similarly, it is not necessary to use an MDSS to determine when to use acetaminophen or ibuprofen for the symptomatic relief of a simple headache.

There are several general classes of medical decision-support systems, including reminder systems, consultation systems, and educational systems. The criteria for the appropriate use of each type of MDSS vary.

Reminder systems

Reminder systems are data-driven. Certain events, such as the ordering of a medication, the appearance of a patient in a clinic for a scheduled visit, or the advent of a particular time of year (e.g., influenza season) trigger activation of reminders that direct health care practitioners' attention to clinical guidelines or possible adverse events regarding patient care. McDonald, Tierney, and their colleagues at the Regenstreif Institute of Indiana University Medical Center have shown through careful studies that physicians are too busy to deliver the care that they readily know is optimal – and that computer-based reminder systems can help them to improve that level of care (McDonald 1976; McDonald et al. 1984; Tierney, Miller, and McDonald 1990; McDonald, Hui, and Tierney 1992). Similarly, Classen, Gardner, and their colleagues at LDS Hospital associated with the University of Utah have shown that reminder systems for ordering of prophylactic antibiotics before surgery can substantially reduce postoperative infections by insuring that all eligible patients receive the recommended therapy in a timely manner (Classen et al. 1992; cf. Larsen et al. 1989; Pestotnik et al. 1990; Evans et al. 1991; Evans et al. 1992; Evans et al. 1993; Evans et al. 1994).

The implementation of a reminder system requires the availability of at least a partial electronic medical record system. For that reason, the impact of such systems in inpatient and, especially, outpatient settings is currently limited. Nevertheless, opportunities for implementation of useful reminder systems are available today. Most pharmacies in the United States, for instance, have prescription registration and monitoring software. It is therefore possible to use reminder systems to prevent administration of medications to which the patient has a past history of allergic reactions, and to notify prescribers when a patient's medications may interact in a potentially dangerous manner.

Literally thousands of clinical guidelines have been generated by reputable organizations (the U.S. Agency for Health Care Policy and Research, National Institutes of Health consensus panels, and professional societies such as the American College of Physicians; and European counterparts), in addition to those published in the peer-reviewed literature and those developed in various locales by groups of regional health care practitioners. It has often been suggested that in clinical medicine, there are more exceptions than rules. A major ethical concern is whether the guidelines developed at one time by one group of individuals for a particular class of patients are relevant to all patients at all times in all settings (see Chapter 7). Failure to review guidelines for appropriateness over time can be harmful. While controlled studies have clearly documented the benefits and potential cost savings that properly applied reminder systems can engender, the current pressures of managed care may promote situations in which "standard medical care" is delivered inappropriately to nonstandard individual patients through automated reminder systems. Very few of the thousands of guidelines in existence have been validated through careful clinical trials. To be fair, one must note that the utility of the stethoscope was not validated through such trials before its use became widespread, either. A certain amount of common sense is required.

The key to the success of reminder systems is their signal-to-noise ratio.

If busy health care practitioners receive what they perceive to be too many "false" or "irrelevant" alarms for every useful suggestion generated by a reminder system, they may ignore all reminders, and so risk harm to patients. Conversely, unless enough information about each patient is available in the electronic medical record to detect when exceptions to general rules apply, the clinician may be persuaded to act inappropriately 5 percent of the time by a system that gives good advice 95 percent of the time. Important considerations are, therefore, these:

- Which guidelines should be used in a given clinical practice setting and for a particular patient?
- Who should decide which guidelines to implement in a particular environment (the practitioner, the government, or the institutional review board)?
- When and how should guidelines be reviewed for updating, replacement, or discontinuation?

The policy of evaluating systems in the contexts in which they are used thus emerges as an overarching practical and ethical requirement (see Chapter 5). This is to point out only that *information* is often vital to identifying ethically optimal decisions.

Concern about "cookbook" medicine or nursing is emblematic of computational progress in all science and industry. Biologists, pilots, mathematicians, and factory-floor managers may all mourn the days before computers and automation, but the ultimate criterion for any new technology is this: Will it serve us better? In health care the question is, Will it improve patient and community well-being? If so, then, all other things being equal, we should use it. That this is a very difficult question to answer is a scientific matter, not an ethical one. That we must make ethical decisions in the face of scientific uncertainty has always been one of the great challenges for clinicians.

Consultation systems

Another model for MDSS use is as a consultant. A consultant system captures or represents medical expertise either on a class of problems (e.g., diagnosis in internal medicine [Miller 1994]) or for a specific problem (such as interpretation of electrocardiograms [Willems et al. 1991], or detection of breast masses and clustered microcalcifications [Nishikawa et al. 1995], or prescription of the most appropriate antibiotic for a given infection [Shortliffe 1976]). The user must determine when it is appropriate to consult such a system, just as a health care provider now determines when it is appropriate to make a referral to a specialist. With current managed care initiatives encouraging fewer referrals and greater emphasis on primary care, a key concern is whether consultant systems can play a constructive role by reducing the need for expert consultant opinions, or whether faulty advice from consultant programs will not be recognized as faulty by primary caregivers who have less contact with specialists than in the past. The complementary viewpoint is also possible, though less likely: Use of expert systems may actually *increase* referrals to specialists, because difficult cases may be more readily identified as such by primary care givers who have access to additional expertise.

One ethical issue regarding use of expert consultation programs is related to the state of their medical knowledge, and their overall validity and accuracy. Massive amounts of effort are required to build and maintain the medical knowledge bases used by consultation systems (Giuse et al. 1989; Musen and van der Lei 1989; Miller and Giuse 1991). If persons not qualified to do so are engaged in such activities, or if timely updating is not performed, the user (and ultimately the patient) may suffer from inappropriate advice. There are no existing standards for "continuing medical education" credits for consultation systems, even though there are such standards for health care providers. For this reason, one must be wary of a medical consultation system's advice, even with a program that has been evaluated in a controlled trial and shown to be valid, if more than a year or two has passed since that trial.

A related point is that there remain exciting and unsettled scientific and conceptual questions about the best way to represent medical knowledge, and, indeed, whether a knowledge representation or an artificial intelligence approach is superior to a statistical method. Scientific differences that shape approaches to system design must be considered in any evaluation of the propriety of using a computer for decision support.

Here is another way to articulate this important ethical concern: Uncertainty about a tool's accuracy and reliability requires cautious use of the tool. This is true for screwdrivers and scalpels alike. When the tool is used in patient care, then morality requires that such caution be assigned the highest possible priority.

A second concern regarding the use of consultation programs involves the imperfect nature of human-machine interaction. There are no guarantees that a system "understands" the information the user inputs into the program, even when the behavior of the program seems to be appropriate for the situation. Similarly, there are no guarantees that the user will understand what a given MDSS output message was intended to mean by the system developers. Lack of standardized medical terms, vocabularies, and definitions leads to confusion among humans, as well as between humans and machines. Harm to patients can result from the faulty interpretation of man-machine communications in either direction. There are few, if any, ancillary clues of the sort used by humans in face-to-face verbal communication (e.g., puzzled facial expression, quizzical tone of voice, nervous tic) to indicate that something may not be ''right'' about the information conveyed. Even greater risks will occur when the source of the patient information is not the primary care provider but, instead, the electronic medical record, since only program-to-program communication will be required to convey a case history to a consultation program for analysis.

Educational systems

Construction of MDSS knowledge bases can be educational for students in the health professions (Miller and Schaffner 1982; Lee, Cutts, Sharp, and Mitchell 1987; Giuse, Giuse, and Miller 1989; Miller and Masarie 1989). The process involves critical review and synthesis of the medical literature and comparison with expert clinicians' opinions, as well as gaining familiarity with bibliographic searching programs and decision-support systems. A number of groups have used medical decision-support systems in the context of teaching problem-solving strategies to medical students. It is also likely that construction of MDSS knowledge bases can identify areas where little is known (such as the findings on urinalysis of patients with legionella infections), and where further clinical studies may be of value.

  A key concern is the viewpoint promoted by many educators that once we have easy access to knowledge via computer databases, it will not be necessary to cram future medical (and other health professional) students' minds full of facts that they will forget anyway – freeing up time to teach a more humanistic and logical approach to patients and medical care. While this perspective seems attractive at first pass, it is not clear that ultimate good would result from such an educational strategy. The ability to detect or recognize a condition (such as a disease state or symptom) depends on one's knowing about that condition or symptom. If all knowledge is relegated to computer data banks, then the ability of the practitioner to recognize any but the most common disorders will diminish over time (a well-known phenomenon: Busy physicians engaged in medical practice, especially if they are isolated from academic medical centers and other colleagues, "lose touch" with the state of the art in diagnosis and therapy beginning about 5 to 10 years after receiving their M.D. degrees). The converse argument has merit, however. If physicians regularly access computer-based information on the diseases of their patients, they will, in a relatively painless and particularly relevant manner, be continually updated regarding the state of the art.

Anecdotally, one of the authors of this chapter (Randolph A. Miller) has been told by a number of clinicians that the use of a medical decision-support system can lead even seasoned clinicians to develop altered, new, and improved approaches to medical problem-solving, even in the subsequent absence of the system. A key concern, however, is whether prolonged use of MDSS, and reliance on them, will lead to clinicians who are more self-sufficient and better educated through exposure to materials they might not otherwise encounter, or whether use of MDSS will in the long term create more passive and dependent and less knowledgeable clinicians. If such skill degradation occurs, it should be considered in the overall decision about the value of deploying such systems.

These are empirical questions, but with no or few answers. Decision making in contexts marked by uncertainty is frequently a rich source of ethical conflict and controversy. When consequences cannot be predicted with any confidence or accuracy, one loses a powerful tool for ethical analysis. In such contexts, caution – neither boosterism nor primitivism – is the appropriate course.

How to – and who should – use a decision-support system

The stethoscope, by itself, is inert. Like other tools, it requires a trained user, and it should not be used without a proper understanding of patient care and the individual patient's case. It must be possible for the user to interpret and even override the data generated through the use of any clinically relevant tool, including a decision-support system.

When a practitioner uses such a system, several ethical concerns may arise. First, there is a question of the user's qualifications. Just as managed care has fueled debates among groups of health care providers about who is qualified, or best qualified, to deliver primary care (physicians, nurse practitioners, physician assistants, social workers, and others), the ethical requirement that the user of a system must be able to recognize potentially faulty advice – a standard imposed by the legal community on physicians when they seek a human consultant's opinion – may spark further debates.

On the other hand, it may be possible, through the use of consultation programs, to enhance the performance of nurse practitioners and of physician assistants to the level of primary care physicians (who have more training). It is clear that whichever viewpoint prevails, the primary caregiver will need to understand the human condition as well as be able to use computer systems (Miller and Giuse 1991). Studies will be required to determine the safety and efficacy of consultation programs in the hands of different classes of users. (Note in this regard the emerging literature comparing accuracy and performance of different systems [Berner et al. 1994].)

Apart from training in clinical practice, a second serious ethical concern emerges from questions about the level of training in the use of computer decision-support systems themselves. A major shortcoming of almost all advanced programs for diagnostic and/or therapeutic consultation currently in the marketplace is the lack of high-quality end-user training. Novice MDSS users have different mindsets than envisioned by system developers, and they imagine such systems to have abilities which, in fact, they do not. For this reason, novice users may try to use MDSS in inappropriate situations. Conversely, novice users might not realize that certain functions built into a decision-support program are even possible. Without proper training, such users would fail to employ a system in situations where it could provide significant benefit. It is unethical for general internists to perform surgery routinely or to perform procedures normally requiring subspecialty certification (such as gastrointestinal endoscopy or cardiac catheterization). It is similarly unethical for general surgeons to routinely perform neurosurgical procedures when a competent neurosurgeon is available. Why should it be considered ethical (or at least common practice, as at the present time) to allow novice, untrained users of sophisticated consultant programs to use them in routine patient care without first demonstrating proficiency, or at least taking certified training courses?

Put differently: The use of decision-support systems in medicine, nursing, and psychology (and for that matter in manufacturing, testing, finance, and so forth) entails responsibilities that are best met by establishing and adhering to educational standards. The ethical imperative is clear in the health professions, and it mirrors the idea of a clinical standard of care. Good intentions, curiosity, and a little knowledge are insufficient to the practice of medicine and nursing. A standard of care embodies the idea of publicly evaluated criteria for decision making and procedural aptitude. There is no reason to suppose that use of decision-support machines should be exempt from such criteria.

The professional-patient relationship

Professionals and lay people tend to have well-focused ideas about what constitutes the proper physician- or provider-patient relationship. In the modern era, we can identify one powerful trend by pointing to Osler (1932) and the idea of the physician as servant to humanity. More recently it has been compellingly suggested that the relationship is most properly understood as a fiduciary one, or one based on compassion, or benevolence and trust. (See for instance Brody 1988; Pellegrino and Thomasma 1988. The fiduciary model is also the standard model in law. Note that other models, emphasizing covenants, contracts, and other relationships, have also been defended.) This depiction of the relationship is not a nicety, a courtesy, a bromide for students suffering moral discomfort or requiring an antidote to hubris. It is the embodiment of values that give structure to interactions in which the knowing and powerful come to the aid of the ignorant and vulnerable.

The decisions a physician or nurse or psychologist makes are customarily made *within* that relationship. On a case-by-case basis, the decisions can even shape the relationship: to test for an incurable disease; to trade, through drug therapy, hypertension for impotence; to warn of risks that might or might not be acceptable because of reasons never expressed and biology not clearly understood. Indeed, the very idea that decisions are made *by* physicians *for* patients is itself being supplanted by the more robust notion of "shared decision making" (Forrow, Wartman, and Brock 1988).

What kind of role can and should a machine play against this backdrop? We might of course just reject the idea of a special physician-patient relationship as feckless feel-goodism that should not impede technological prospects for better outcomes. In this case, the machine's role could be extensive. We might even contemplate a machine replacing a human altogether. But this is spurious.

What is wrong is that the practice of medicine or nursing is not exclusively and clearly scientific, statistical, or procedural, and hence is not, so far, computationally tractable. This is not to make a hoary appeal to the "art and science" of medicine; it is to say that the science is in many contexts inadequate or inapplicable: Many clinical decisions are not exclusively medical – they have social, personal, ethical, psychological, financial, familial, legal, and other components; even art might play a role. While we should be thrilled to behold the machine that will make these decisions correctly – at least pass a medical Turing test – a more sober course is to acknowledge that, for the present at least, human physicians and nurses make the best clinical decisions. This entails ethical obligations of the sort identified here.

There is a further question: To what extent do *patients* need to understand decision-support systems before their consent to machine-mediated decisions, procedures, or interventions can be considered informed? Not only is the best answer to this question unknown, it is not yet clear what would constitute an acceptable range of answers. (The question of informed or valid consent in this context would constitute an interesting and worthwhile area for research to complement investigations aimed at learning about professional attitudes toward health computing.) The point is that patients now have at least some notion of what is involved in human decision making. With robust and increasingly accurate decision-support systems, those conceptions become outdated. Should patients be told the accuracy rate of decision machines – when they never were given comparable data for humans? Would knowledge of such rates maximize the validity of consent, or constitute another befuddling ratio that inspires doubt more than it informs rationality? (See Chapter 8 for a discussion of sharing computational mortality predictions with patients and families.)

The decisions one makes in medical, nursing, and psychology clinics have consequences. Computational decision support has consequences, too. In the context of physician-patient and other professional-patient relationships, one must weigh the risk of eroded trust from using a tool sometimes seen as occult against the risk of failing to employ decision support where it could improve treatment. Seeking such a balance constitutes the kind of challenge which advances in medical technology have presented, repeatedly, for millennia.

Conclusion

The use of medical decision-support systems will continue to increase as computers are improved, as users become more sophisticated, and as socioeconomic factors demand such an increase. Not all such uses will be appropriate; one is duty-bound to select the correct tool for a job, and even appropriate uses must be evaluated against a complex web of reasonable expectations, publicly defensible standards, and rigorous evaluation metrics. It is possible to err here, and err badly.

A robust concern for ethics in practice is not satisfied by stipulating in advance the circumstances in which a particular action would be identified as blameworthy or praiseworthy. Rather, practitioners should have access to a set of moral, professional, and social touchstones by which to find the way. The use of decision-support systems in clinical practice offers ever-increasing promise for improving patient care in a broad variety of settings. But this promise is betrayed if we stray from standards for appropriate tool use, for instance, or when we allow socially productive and respectful relationships to be sullied, or their participants to be taken advantage of.

Fortunately, in medicine, nursing, and many other professions, we knew that already.

References

Berner, E.S., Webster, G.D., Shugerman, A.A., Jackson, J.R., Algina, J., Baker, A.L., Ball, E.V., Cobbs, C.G., Dennis, V.W., Frenkel, E.P., et al. 1994. Performance of four computer-based diagnostic systems. *New England Journal of Medicine* 330: 1792–6.

Brody, B.A. 1988. *Life and Death Decision Making*. New York: Oxford University Press.

Classen, D.C., Evans, R.S., Pestotnik, S.L., Horn, S.D., Menlove, R.L., and Burke, J.P. 1992. The timing of prophylactic administration of antibiotics and the risk of surgical-wound infection. *New England Journal of Medicine* 326: 281–6.

Covell, D.G., Uman, G.C., and Manning, P.R. 1985. Information needs in office practice: Are they being met? *Annals of Internal Medicine* 103: 596–9.

Evans, R.S., Burke, J.P., Classen, D.C., Gardner, R.M., Menlove, R.L., Goodrich, K.M., Stevens, L.E., and Pestotnik, S.L. 1992. Computerized identification of patients at high risk for hospital-acquired infection. *American Journal of Infection Control* 20: 4–10.

Evans, R.S., Classen, D.C., Pestotnik, S.L., Lundsgaarde, H.P., and Burke, J.P. 1994. Improving empiric antibiotic selection using computer decision support. *Archives of Internal Medicine* 154: 878–84.

Evans, R.S., Classen, D.C., Stevens, L.E., Pestotnik, S.L., Gardner, R.M., Lloyd, J.F., and Burke, J.P. 1993. Using a hospital information system to assess the effects of adverse drug events. In *Proceedings of the Seventeenth Annual Symposium on Computer Applications in Medical Care,* ed. C. Safran, pp. 161–5. New York: McGraw-Hill.

Evans, R.S., Pestotnik, S.L., Classen, D.C., Bass, S.B., Menlove, R.L., Gardner, R.M., and Burke, J.P. 1991. Development of a computerized adverse drug event monitor. In *Proceedings of the Fifteenth Annual Symposium on Computer Applications in Medical Care,* ed. P.D. Clayton, pp. 23–7. New York: McGraw-Hill.

Forrow, L., Wartman, S.A., and Brock, D.W. 1988. Science, ethics, and the making of clinical decisions. *Journal of the American Medical Association* 259: 3161–7.

Giuse, N.B., Bankowitz, R.A., Giuse, D.A., Parker, R.C., and Miller, R.A. 1989. Medical knowledge base acquisition: the role of expert review process in disease profile construction. In *Proceedings of the Thirteenth Annual Symposium on Computer Applications in Medical Care,* ed. L.C. Kingsland, pp. 105–9. Washington, D.C.: IEEE Computer Society Press.

Giuse, N.B., Giuse, D.A., and Miller, R.A. 1989. Medical knowledge base construction as a means of introducing students to medical informatics. In *Proceedings of the Thirteenth Annual Symposium on Computer Applications in Medical Care,* ed. L.C. Kingsland, pp. 228–32. Washington, D.C.: IEEE Computer Society Press.

Larsen, R.A., Evans, R.S., Burke, J.P., Pestotnik, S.L., Gardner, R.M., and Classen, D.C. 1989. Improved perioperative antibiotic use and reduced surgical wound infections through use of computer decision analysis. *Infection Control and Hospital Epidemiology* 10: 316–20.

Lee, A.S., Cutts, J.H., Sharp, G.C., and Mitchell, J.A. 1987. AI/LEARN network: The use of computer-generated graphics to augment the educational utility of a knowledge-based diagnostic system (AI/RHEUM). *Journal of Medical Systems* 11: 349–58.

McDonald, C.J. 1976. Protocol-based computer reminders, the quality of care and the non-perfectibility of man. *New England Journal of Medicine* 295: 1351–5.

McDonald, C.J., Hui, S.L., Smith, D.M., et al. 1984. Reminders to physicians from an introspective computer medical record. *Annals of Internal Medicine* 100: 130–8.

McDonald, C.J., Hui, S.L., and Tierney, W.M. 1992. Effects of computer reminders for influenza vaccination on morbidity during influenza epidemics. *MD Computing* 9: 304–12.

Miller, R.A. 1990. Why the standard view is standard: People, not machines, understand patients' problems. *Journal of Medicine and Philosophy* 15: 581–91.

Miller, R.A. 1994. Medical diagnostic decision-support systems – past, present, and future: a threaded bibliography and commentary. *Journal of the American Medical Informatics Association* 1: 8–27.

Miller, R.A., and Giuse, N.B. 1991. Medical knowledge bases. *Academic Medicine* 66:15–17.

Miller, R.A., and Masarie, F.E. 1989. Use of the Quick Medical Reference (QMR) program as a tool for medical education. *Methods of Information in Medicine* 28: 340–5.

Miller, R.A., and Schaffner, K.F. 1982. The logic of problem-solving in clinical diagnosis: a course for second-year medical students. *Journal of Medical Education* 57: 63–5.

Miller, R.A., Schaffner, K.F., and Meisel, A. 1985. Ethical and legal issues related to the use of computer programs in clinical medicine. *Annals of Internal Medicine* 102: 529–36.

Musen, M.A., and van der Lei, J. 1989. Knowledge engineering for clinical consultation programs: modeling the application area. *Methods of Information In Medicine.* 28: 28–35.

Nishikawa, R.M., Haldemann, R.C., Papaioannou, J., Giger, M.L., Lu, P., Schmidt, R.A., Wolverton, D.E., Bick, U., and Doi, K. 1995. Initial experience with a prototype clinical "intelligent" mammography workstation for computer-aided diagnosis. *Proceedings of the Society of Photo-optical Instrumentation Engineering,* pp. 65–71, No. 2434, Bellingham, Wash.: SPIE.

Osheroff, J.A., Forsythe, D.E., Buchanan, B.G., Bankowitz, R.A., Blumenfeld, B.H., and Miller, R.A. 1991 Physicians' information needs: an analysis of questions posed during clinical teaching in internal medicine. *Annals of Internal Medicine* 114: 576–81.

Osler, W. 1932. *Aequanimitas: With other Addresses to Medical Students, Nurses and Practitioners of Medicine,* 3rd ed. Philadelphia: P. Blakiston's Son & Co.

Pellegrino, E.D., and Thomasma, D.C. 1988. *For the Patient's Good: The Restoration of Beneficence in Health Care.* New York: Oxford University Press.

Pestotnik, S.L., Evans, R.S., Burke, J.P., Gardner, R.M., and Classen, D.C. 1990. Therapeutic antibiotic monitoring: surveillance using a computerized expert system. *American Journal of Medicine* 88: 43–8.

Shortliffe, E.H. 1976. *Computer-Based Medical Consultations: MYCIN.* New York: Elsevier/North Holland.

Shortliffe, E.H. 1987. Computer programs to support clinical decision making. *Journal of the American Medical Association* 258: 61–6.

Tierney, W.M., Miller, M.E., and McDonald, C.J. 1990. The effect on test ordering of informing physicians of the charges for outpatient diagnostic tests. *New England Journal of Medicine* 322: 1499–504.

Willems, J.L., Abreu-Lima, C., Arnaud, P., van Bemmel, J.H., Brohet, C., Degani, R., Denis, B., Gehring, J., Graham, I., van Herpen, G., et al. 1991. The diagnostic performance of computer programs for the interpretation of electrocardiograms. *New England Journal of Medicine* 325: 1767–73.

7

Outcomes, futility, and health policy research
KENNETH W. GOODMAN

If only they could predict the future, health professionals would know in advance who will live, who will die, and who will benefit from this or that treatment, drug, or procedure. Foreknowledge would come in very handy indeed in hospitals and, in fact, has been a goal of medicine since antiquity. Computers dramatically improve our ability to calculate how things will turn out. This means we can use them in clinical decision making and, at the other end of the health care spectrum, in deciding which policy, method, or budget will produce the desired results. This chapter takes as its starting point the use of prognostic scoring systems in critical care and reviews their applications and limitations. It concludes that such systems are inadequate in themselves for identifying instances of clinical futility, in part because it is not logically appropriate to apply outcome scores to individual patients; such scores should be regarded as a point in an evidentiary constellation, and should not alone be allowed to defeat other considerations in the care of critically ill patients. Similarly, the rapid increase in the use of computers to derive practice guidelines across the health care spectrum represents an important extension of requirements that decisions be informed by the best available evidence. But computers cannot determine whether guidelines are applicable in individual cases, or develop guidelines that are. These, like other tasks in health care, belong to humans, especially when resource allocation is at stake.

Introduction

In the curious opening section of his *Prognosis* Hippocrates suggests: "One must know to what extent [diseases] exceed the strength of the body and one must have a thorough acquaintance with their future course. In this way one may become a good physician and justly win high fame. In

Parts of this chapter appeared in Goodman (1996) and are adapted and revised here with the permission of W.B. Saunders Company. I am grateful to Dr. Kathryn Koch for comments on an earlier version.

116

the case of patients who were going to survive, he would be able to safeguard them the better from complications by having a longer time to take precautions. By realizing and announcing beforehand which patients were going to die, [the physician] would absolve himself from any blame'' (Hippocrates 1983:170). In other words, one of the values of an accurate medical prediction is improved marketing and public relations!

More than two millennia later, the ability to predict the course of an illness continues to have social and economic value. And it still has public relations value, at least to the extent that managed competition is driven by health care providers who compete for patients on the basis of public reports of outcomes and cost.

Outcome predictions, practice guidelines, evidence-based medicine, and the like are the new engines of health care, at least in Europe and North America. These engines are computational. This chapter examines the role of computers in making medical predictions. Because the evolution of prognostic scoring systems in critical care raises such keen ethical issues, these systems will be emphasized here. Findings about such systems will generally be applicable to related but distinct uses of computers to render prognoses or calculate outcomes. Some of those issues will be considered here, and some in Chapter 8.

Computing and prognosis

The logic and structure of scientific prediction raise some of the oldest, most interesting, and most difficult problems in the philosophy of science. Prediction is bound up with the logics of induction and deduction, the problem of scientific explanation, issues in confirmation, the problem of determinism, and the role of causation. There is nothing about medical predictions that insulates them from these conceptual and philosophical concerns. Now, medical predictions, or, sometimes, *prognoses*, are especially important to humans. They chart the future course of our illnesses; they discourage us or give us hope; and occasionally they tell us how long we've got. The melodramatic inquiry, ''What are my chances, Doc?'' is a demand for a prediction. It is always a probabilistic prediction, even though we sometimes reckon the probability to be quite high, or low.

Prognostic scoring systems

For nearly two decades, researchers have been working to develop computer programs and databases that will enable them to estimate the short-term mortality for intensive care patients. In other words, many illness-severity systems predict the likelihood of patients' dying (see Kollef and Schuster 1994 for a scientific and conceptual survey). The best-known of these systems is the APACHE series, where the term is an acronym from "acute physiology, age, chronic health evaluation." The system's origins are traced to the early 1970s when hospitals began routinely to monitor acute physiologic abnormalities (Knaus, Wagner, and Lynn 1991.) By tracking a patient's (1) physiologic data, including variables ranging from blood pressure and serum sodium to blood urea nitrogen and Glasgow Coma Score; (2) demographic characteristics, including where ICU patients are transferred from (emergency department, operating room, etc.); and (3) diagnosis (AIDS, liver failure, metastatic cancer, etc.), the system can compare individual patients to some 20,000 others whose physiologic profiles are maintained in the core database. The patients are assigned a score which represents how much they are like the others, whose demises are known. The higher the score, the greater the likelihood the patient will not survive the hospitalization (see, e.g., Knaus et al. 1991). APACHE-III is a proprietary system that costs about $300,000. Versions have been installed in more than 300 hospitals around the world.

Important alternatives to APACHE include the Mortality Probability Model (MPM) (Lemeshow, Teres, Avrunin, and Gage 1988; Lemeshow et al. 1993); and the Simplified Acute Physiology Score (SAPS) (Le Gall, Lemeshow, and Saulnier 1993).

There are also a number of systems designed for pediatric cases, a domain in which predicting outcomes, especially longer-term outcomes, is especially difficult (Pollack, Ruttimann, and Getson 1988; Ruttimann and Pollack 1991).

Evaluations and comparisons of the different systems have tended to show that mortality probability estimates have fair sensitivity and specificity; misclassification rates range from 10 to 25 percent (Schafer et al. 1990; Castella, Gilabert, Torner, and Torres 1991; Kollef and Schuster 1994; Castella, Artigas, Bion, and Kari 1995). It is important to note that these are very short term measures, usually valid for no more than a week. Moreover, the level of accuracy is itself the topic of some debate. In fact, scientific and methodological disputes over prognostic scoring systems represent a fascinating source of heated medical controversy, and APACHE's designers and others have offered strong defenses of the system's accuracy (Watts and Knaus 1994a, b, c). We will return to questions of error and accuracy below.

Prognostic scoring systems may in any case be best suited for analyzing treatment patterns, for comparing one's institution to others or to itself over time, and thus for evaluating performance – although even these functions are scientifically controversial.

Now, anyone who suggests that medical prediction is easy does not understand it very well. This is perhaps especially true for critical care outcomes, a subset of medical predictions. Several factors contribute to this difficulty:

One, already noted, is conceptual or epistemological. To induce that a particular patient will not survive the week, for instance, is often to presume the reliability of induction, which, while psychologically compelling, raises difficult problems about causation and the role of causation in prognosis.

A second is empirical. Even if we solve the problem of induction we must identify some reliability metric for evaluating the data and statistical tools that drive our inductions. Another way of putting this is in terms of accuracy: Some prediction machines are just not as accurate as we would like, or should insist on.

A third source of difficulty in predicting critical care outcomes is perhaps best described as social: We *use* this information for a variety of social and economic goals. The difficulty here is the temptation to solve a social problem – allocation of resources, say – at an individual patient's bedside. The problem is not in predicting an outcome, but in appropriate use of the prediction.

All three factors raise ethical issues.

Induction and causation

The problem of induction is exciting and difficult. It is no mere philosophical curiosity, but a direct challenge to common ways of increasing knowledge and understanding of the physical world. The problem was first articulated clearly by the 18th-century philosopher David Hume. It is this, more or less: Our inclination to infer causal relations between successive events is *psychological* and not logical. Hume argued that the regular pairing of successive events is not any sort of evidence of a causal relation but, rather, a mere ''constant conjunction'' (Hume 1969). Pairings of events reveal only that the second event followed the first, not that it was caused by it. This is the case for collisions of billiard balls, motions of the planets, and courses of disease. It does not matter how many times we observe the pairing – we still lack grounds for belief in a causal connection, Hume argued. (A favorite example among philosophers to illustrate this point goes something like this: "Every time I get a cold I retreat to my barn and swing a chicken around my head three times. Without fail, in two weeks' time the cold is gone.")

Hume's skepticism has been a popular target for generations of thinkers. Whether the problem of induction has been solved is a matter of some controversy. The point for our purposes can be simply put: To say that a patient will not live another week, in light of the fact that most other patients like him have not lived a week, is to infer inductively from past cases to the future of the current case – it is not to say that we have identified the causal mechanism that will lead to his death; neither is it to say that we can predict the *cause* of his death.

Skepticism, it should be argued, is an unhappy and wrongheaded stance toward the possibility of scientific knowledge, Hume notwithstanding. As medical science advances it acquires truths about the human organism. Eventually we acquire knowledge by stronger, deductive, means (although we must acknowledge that some deductions are made possible by inductive establishment of general rules). In the modern era and the current context, Hume's challenge is best understood as telling us not that we cannot learn about the causal course of illness or trauma, but that we must be on guard against over-facile predictions. We must resist the temptation to assume closure for any individual patient because of the weight of previous experiences with other patients. Notice that there is no contradiction between this proviso and the observation that we do in fact learn from such previous experiences.

Consider in this regard the fact that most critical care scoring systems are, like human judgment, statistical and probabilistic. The question for clinicians is as follows. In the absence of certainty about the course of an individual patient's hospitalization, when and to what degree is it appropriate to rely on statistical metrics for decision making? We still have no good answer to this question. The development of probabilistic models that attempt to quantify illness severity is a good way to attempt to respond to clinical uncertainty (Ruttimann 1994). But challenges in selecting predictor variables are substantial, and progress here must await progress in the science of statistics itself: "The hope is that progress in statistical methodology gradually will replace some of the currently used ad hoc approaches with more objective procedures" (Ruttimann 1994: 22).

Clinical judgment is a precious touchstone in medical and nursing decision making. But what is the gold standard for validating clinical judgment? Is clinical judgment not based on the past experiences of the clinician and his or her teachers? That is, much clinical judgment itself is statistically – inductively – driven. Also, individual human judgments are in principle subject to error and bias, which are among the very properties that have inspired the growth of medical computing in the first place. In some respects, this is just the distinction between subjective and objective probability estimates (Knaus, Wagner, and Lynn 1991). The clinician's prediction is subjective; the computer's is objective. Nevertheless, mature clinical decision making relies on more than data and inference. The experienced practitioner knows that many key clinical decisions are successful because they take patient values and needs into account; this is not a computable skill.

Here is where we stand so far: (1) Statistical methods cannot eliminate uncertainty; (2) methods of reducing uncertainty require further development; and (3) clinical judgment may serve as a check on computer-mediated predictions (and vice versa), but these judgments themselves are not immune to uncertainty, and are subject to error and bias.

Error and accuracy

There is a great deal we do not know about medical outcomes. We do not know all the ways of calculating them, or the best way to predict them, or what effects their reporting has on patients, families, and professional colleagues. We have a long way to go in developing evaluation metrics for medical prediction machines and, in statistics, in validating predictor models. We are faced with a comparatively new science, and it is in ferment. In the context of critical care, there are by one count at least 20 different illness-severity scoring systems (Vassar and Holcroft 1994), and, as noted earlier, proponents of different systems are competing intensively.

Consider the need for system evaluation. If one were going to evaluate the quality of a scoring system one might compare it to (1) other scoring systems, (2) human experts, (3) local outcomes, (4) other sets of outcomes, and (5) other prognostic tools. These comparison points are distinct from some criteria or requirements identified as necessary for developing scoring systems in the first place (Vassar and Holcroft 1994). But tests of noncausal accuracy are mere parlor games when it comes to evaluating the efficacy of clinical tools. If we cannot say why a particular outcome or intervention will occur, but only that we are more or less confident it will occur given certain antecedent conditions, then we have given away one of our most precious tools for explaining and understanding the world.

The crucial question is this: Can computer software that predicts outcomes be used to predict outcomes in individual cases? The question cannot be answered independently of evidence about the accuracy of the predictions. Critical care scoring systems have been criticized for a variety of scientific reasons, including sensitivity, specificity, predictive value, and ability to contain costs (Civetta 1990; Civetta, Hudson-Civetta, and Nelson 1990; Schafer et al. 1990; Civetta 1991; Teres 1993; Cowen and Kelley 1994; Teres and Lemeshow 1994; Vassar and Holcroft 1994; Iezzoni et al. 1995). The best conclusion is that such software is not accurate enough to warrant or justify use in individual cases. A number of consequences of ethical import follow from this, most notably that decisions to withhold or terminate treatment are problematic if based on a mortality prediction score.

This and related ideas have been near the core of two previous and important efforts to address ethical issues related to the use of prognostic scoring systems (Brody 1989; Luce and Wachter 1994). Thus, ''Our real fear is not that we won't be able to identify in advance all non-survivors, but rather that we will prospectively classify as non-survivors those who would actually survive with good ICU care'' (Brody 1989: 669).

Another way of putting this is as follows: While prognostic scoring systems are very accurate for certain patients in the short term, it is by no means evident what level of accuracy is acceptable *tout court*. Since what is being predicted is no mere medical intervention outcome, but death, the stakes in determining that level of accuracy are very high indeed.

This is not the place to try to resolve this important and exciting debate. Fortunately no such resolution is needed here. The very fact that there is a scientific dispute helps make the following point: In the absence of consensus on use of a new medical tool, we should use such a tool only with the greatest caution, or not at all. The point is grounded in common sense and prudence, not Luddism. Indeed, there might be an *obligation* to develop, test, and use such a tool, if doing so will (eventually) improve patient care or, perhaps, conserve resources in appropriate ways. If it were otherwise, the health sciences could not progress ethically.

It is emphatically not being suggested either that we must be skeptics when it comes to intensive care predictions, or that certainty is a require-ment for sound decision making. Yet uncertainty and indeterminacy are unavoidable features of critical care (and other medical) decisions, no mat-ter what our computational support may be. This is not an argument against using new scoring tools, but an insistence that we understand their limitations and resist the temptation to assume that computer output pro-vides a scientifically privileged view of clinical outcomes. It is an argu-ment for caution. It is an argument in favor of more and better analyses of the appropriate contexts of use of predictive scoring systems. These points may be seen as ethical imperatives.

Social utility of predictor models

Computational futility metrics

We have been discussing reasons why it is difficult to predict critical care outcomes. We now need to address the question of what to do with a prediction if we believe it to be (more or less) accurate.

At their best, critical care scoring systems are supposed to provide us with an objective way to identify for individual patients at least one aspect of medical futility. Let us define a "computational futility metric" (CFM) as any prognostic scoring system output that purports to demonstrate that future treatment will produce no benefit on at least one axis of a well-known typology of clinical goals (Youngner 1988).

- Physiological: e.g., when catecholamines do not increase blood pressure
- Postponing death: when intervention will not prolong life
- Length of life: when a life is saved, but only for a short while
- Quality of life: when life is prolonged but not improved
- Probability of success: when there is small chance of prolonging life, or prolonging life with quality

What makes this typology useful is its demonstration that futility is not a global or monolithic concept, that decisions about further treatment must be relativized to goals (Youngner 1988). Additionally, there are rival models of physician obligations in futile or purportedly futile contexts (Jecker and Schneiderman 1993; Schneiderman and Jecker 1995). Under the weak model, physicians are free to withhold or discontinue futile efforts; a moderate obligation has it that physicians should be encouraged to withhold or discontinue futile efforts; in the strong model, physicians must withhold or discontinue futile efforts. Each model has various strengths and weaknesses. What such a typology suggests is that there is much work to be done – independently of outcomes accuracy and prognostic scoring – before we can proclaim that a CFM provides support for terminating or withholding treatment (cf. Luce and Wachter 1994). This effort will occur in bioethics and related disciplines, where, it must be strongly emphasized, debates about futility are intense, multidisciplinary, and waged on many fronts. We have no uniform definition of futility, or even an agreement that one is needed. The idea that a severity score, even an objective one, can help determine whether a case is futile is like trying to take a measurement one day with a meter rod, the next with a yardstick, and the third in cubits – unless the unit of measurement is agreed on, it makes no sense to suggest that yet another measurement will give the true length.

Society needs to decide how to address futility, and what resources it thereby hopes to conserve (Teno et al. 1994). It just will not do for system designers or clinicians to (1) proclaim the accuracy of a particular CFM, (2) appeal to a favorite or favorable position or argument on futility (or any other outcome-related concept), and (3) link the two in such a way as to suggest that further treatment may or must be withheld.

The point has been made in the following way. Scientific data are of no value unless interpreted: "A finding of enzyme level X has no ethical significance in and of itself, even once its prognostic significance has been decided. An ethical judgment must be made about the implications of the prognostic significance in question" (Dagi 1993: 264). Such implications must take into consideration the wishes of competent patients or valid surrogates. Baruch Brody, in a keystone contribution to the ethics of prognostic scoring systems, puts it as follows:

Suppose that, with the help of a validated severity of illness scale, clinicians can accurately estimate the probability of the patient's surviving [the] current hospitalization if he or she receives all interventions available. Is that information as useful as it might seem initially? I think not. Patients who have a very poor probability of surviving their current hospitalization may still obtain through extensive medical interventions a prolongation of their life in the hospital before they die. This prolongation may be judged by them and/or their family to be of considerable significance.

Conversely, patients who have a very high probability of surviving their current hospitalization through extensive interventions, but whose more long-term prognosis (even their six month survival rate) is extremely poor, may judge (or their families may judge for them) that the prolongation of life is of little significance compared to the heavy costs imposed by the extensive interventions. Clinicians who use severity of illness scales to determine the likelihood of survival for the current hospitalization, and who make judgments of futility or of utility on the basis of this likelihood, have chosen as their outcome-measure something that may not correspond either with their patient's values or with their own values (Brody 1989: 663).

This point and its variations have come to be part of a sort of "standard theory" of prognostic scoring systems in critical care. Listen to the developers of the best-known such system: "Objective probability estimates will frequently confirm uncertainty regarding the patient's ability to survive. Sometimes confidence intervals will be too large to encourage reliance on the point estimate. These characteristics and the continuous nature of the estimates must be emphasized, lest objective estimates be misunderstood as decision rules, which might restrict rather than enhance clinical reasoning'' (Knaus, Wagner, and Lynn 1991: 392). And, ''The value inherent in the system is that medical criteria should form the foundation for decision making and that patients' preferences and values should modify the process'' (Knaus 1993: 196; cf. Sasse 1993).

Such a stance is encouraging. We must realize, however, how much ethical flaccidity it allows. To say that judgments of significance may vary, that clinical reasoning might be restricted, that patient values should modify a process – all this might be trifling in the face of financial and social pressures, and the risky belief among practitioners that a computational metric can close the book on clinical futility.

Defining clinical futility

There is in fact a growing body of anecdotal evidence that individual decisions to reduce or terminate treatment are increasingly being driven by prognostic scores, as for instance in the case of the ''patient who belonged to an HMO who had therapy withdrawn because of respiratory, renal, and hepatic dysfunction that was not particularly severe but who had an 80% mortality based on an APACHE II . . . score'' (Sprung, Eidelman, and Pizov 1996: 515).

Something has gone wrong here. Partly it is this: To maintain simultaneously (1) that prognostic scores define futility and (2) that clinicians and patients and families must include personal values in the service of better judgments of the scores' significance is to impose a contradictory and hence conceptually onerous burden.

The suggestion that a severity scoring system can define futility seems to entail the following sort of statement: ''Further treatment of Ms. X is futile because (or in light of the fact that) her prognostic score is y,'' where y is a value such that most other patients with that score did not survive the week (or whatever). But this is not a definition, any more than ''a hemoglobin of 10'' defines the term ''duodenal ulcer.'' Rather, it defines ''anemia,'' and as such is *evidence* for the bleeding ulcer. APACHE and other severity scores are best understood as evidence that can support hypotheses of poor outcomes.

The distinction is important because clinical prognoses are customarily regarded as embodying a number of intuitions about causation. It is not merely that we infer that a particular antecedent event will be followed by a subsequent event, but that the antecedent event has an *etiologic* role in the subsequent one. With hundreds of disease categories and physiologic variables that go into an illness-severity score, it can be very difficult to identify an etiologic relation.

This is not a problem so long as the user of a critical care scoring system is analyzing treatment patterns, conducting institutional comparisons, or evaluating performance. Decisions are often and accurately based on aggregate data that reveal no or flimsy causal relations. It becomes a problem when one needs to make a decision about the care of individual patients. This obligation traditionally and optimally relies on causal hypotheses, background knowledge, and available evidence. Prognosis without causation is fortune telling.

The logical structure and clinical applications of probability and causation are vast enterprises, and they shape vitally important efforts in science and the philosophy of science. What seems to be needed is a practical approach to probability that warrants decisions of the sort that are allegedly enlightened by critical care scoring systems. Absent such an approach, wise clinicians will use these systems for a variety of purposes, including acquisition of evidence regarding the futility of individual cases. They will not allow the systems to trump, or even erode confidence in, sound clinical decisions by knowledgeable and experienced humans.

Should a prognostic score be shared with patients and families?

As computerized scoring systems become more common and familiar, it will become important to know whether and to what extent practitioners should share outcomes data with patients or their surrogates. The force of a report of clinical judgment ("I'm sorry, but I don't think you'll make it") is embedded in mass culture (it is one possible response to the query "What are my chances, Doc?"), and is strongly attached to the authority that accompanies judgments by trusted physicians and nurses. Contrarily, a CFM report ("I am sorry, but the computer has assigned your loved one a very low probability of survival; here are the multivariate physiological variables that were used in computing . . .") enjoys no such status.

In other words, patient and family naiveté and ignorance are the source of numerous existing problems in delivering bad news. Adding technological spin to such reports contributes little if anything to valid consent by patients or surrogates. Note that this is the case *even if the CFM is perfectly and uncontroversially accurate.* At the end of life, being prognostically correct is itself not a sufficient condition for ethically maximized bedside manner and communication (cf. Brody 1989).

The question, ''Should a prognostic score be shared with patients and families?'' actually has two versions: Should the score be reported if it is asked for? and Should it be communicated if it is not requested (including here cases in which patients and families do not even know of the score's existence)?

If patients or their families are sophisticated enough to know about prognostic scoring systems, and they request this information, then it should be given, along with a strong dose of background information and caveats. The disadvantages of playing a numbers game are outweighed by the disadvantages of deception or withholding information, even prognostic scoring information.

If patients or families are ignorant of objective probability estimates, it is probably inappropriate to tell them (unless the information has contributed significantly to any clinical decision or recommendation, which use I am arguing is inappropriate in the first place). Doing so will seem significant when it is not. Actual decisions, however, will need to be planned, scrutinized, and evaluated on a case-by-case basis. It might be appropriate to share a mortality estimate in cases where little or no other data are available, but this is fraught with the same problems that attach to giving patients or families any sort of numerical outcome estimate: These estimates are hard to understand, they carry more weight than they should, and they are only one component of a rich tableau of decision points. The physician or nurse who offers a subjective estimate faces the same problem. If a clinician tells a patient that a cancer is fatal in 90 percent of all cases, where this estimate is based on personal experience or recollection, the utility of this information cannot be evaluated independently of the clinician-patient relationship, the patient's goals and expectations, the margin of error, the basis for the estimate, and so forth. Clinical truth telling requires more than numbers, even objective or accurate numbers, to be of value. One suspects that outcome-scoring software is sometimes eagerly embraced because it is viewed as making a very difficult task – giving bad news – easier. Given the educational component that must accompany any reporting of mortality predictions, such hoped-for ease would be wildly overstated.

Cost containment and resource allocation

The current climate in health care delivery and financing is very queer indeed. CFM's (or related measures) are frequently cited as means of ensuring a just allocation of health resources (Knaus, Wagner, and Lynn 1991; Luce and Wachter 1994). The idea is that an objective measure of futility or medical usefulness will help society deploy scarce critical care resources where they will do the most good, and not squander them where they will not do any good, or do too little.

If I understand this view correctly, it is this: Society's inability to come to terms with death, our collective denial of the dying process, and our refusal to acknowledge when the good fight should be abandoned are all due to a lack of objective *information*. It would be very nice if this were so. But it is not. We have had increasingly accurate information about outcomes for millennia. There is no shortage of evidence that many patients and/or surrogates are inclined to seek a full-court press against death, even in the absence of warrant to believe that it will do any good. The problem in each of these "do everything" cases is not a lack of objective information. It is rather a lack of education, a failure of communication, or a psychological inability to grasp when the game is lost. No CFM, no objective mortality prediction, no computational line in the sand will accomplish what generations of families, physicians, nurses, and patients have failed to accomplish: a broad-based, mature, and realistic view of death and dying. Saddling computerized death predictions with the responsibility for helping solve society's resource allocation problems is like hoping that removing the straw will heal the camel's back.

The following represents a worst-case scenario: A computer score is used as the deciding factor to withdraw or withhold treatment for the sake of cost containment. There is an important, interesting – and conflicting – body of research that tracks the use of do-not-resuscitate orders against cost savings (Emanuel and Emanuel 1994; Rapoport, Teres, and Lemeshow 1996). At the point at which a mortality score or CFM is linked to a purported cost savings, we will have crossed a terrible Rubicon. Worse, that any insurance or managed competition plan would require or reward treatment refusals based solely on a CFM is conditioned on fallacious reasoning, poor understanding, and arrested ethical development.

Practice guidelines

Clinical guidelines are rapidly proliferating on both sides of the Atlantic.
(*Haines and Feder 1992*)

Outcomes research is complete rubbish.
(*Richard Peto, in Computers & Medicine 1994*)

Rules and databases

In remarks on what goes on when people follow rules, the philosopher Ludwig Wittgenstein gives an example similar to the following: A pupil is asked to complete the series of numerals "2, 4, 6, 8, 10 . . ." He continues the series by writing "13, 16, 19." We suggest that the pupil did not understand his instructions, that he got it wrong. But he says that he thought the rule was to increase by 2 up to 10, then by 3, which would constitute a perfectly valid numerical series. What is it, outside of the intention of the questioner, that makes an answer correct? One can imagine clearly that any numeral after 10 could in principle be the next integer in a valid series. Wittgenstein's question is, "How is it decided what is the right step to take at any particular stage?" (Wittgenstein 1968: 75e).

The world does not *intend* for us to understand it correctly. An answer to a scientific or medical question is not correct because we have identified what Nature had in mind. An accurate medical prediction, or an algorithm for making one, is useful as far as it goes. The point here is that sometimes it does not go very far at all.

Still, research on outcomes, practice guidelines, and evidence-based medicine has in a comparatively short time become one of health care's greatest growth industries. Everyone, it seems, now studies outcomes. Governments, professional groups, hospitals, insurance companies, managed care organizations, pharmaceutical companies, employers, and others are collecting data with the idea of monitoring or improving quality, reducing costs, and even rationing, or at least allocating, resources.

Florence Nightingale's proposal more than a century ago to track outcomes has emerged as perhaps the most powerful engine driving health care change, at least in Europe and North America. The fuel for this engine is information, contained in numerous, increasingly interconnected databases. Managed competition is supposed to rely in part precisely on free access to these data.

Wittgenstein's point, in conjunction with the lessons about use of critical care scoring systems, should illuminate a stance, an ethical position, regarding use of outcomes information. Let us look at two broad domains in which ethical issues arise: (1) adequacy, accuracy, and resource allocation; and (2) human subjects research. The upshot of these brief reviews will parallel that of prognostic scoring systems.

Adequacy, accuracy, and resource allocation

The fervor with which new technologies are sometimes embraced is remarkable. In the case of outcomes research, the enthusiasm is understandable: Better evidence makes for better decisions. If an intervention does not work, or does not work very well, then there is no or little point in providing it, or paying for it. Decision making in medicine, nursing, and the other health sciences is based in part on beliefs about efficacy. And so it is important that outcomes research advance. Shooting from the hip, betting on hunches, and taking a stab at it are generally inferior decision procedures. This was the idea a quarter of a century ago when the British epidemiologist Archie Cochrane bemoaned the fact that there was no comprehensive and up-to-date repository of clinical trial results for use by practitioners (Cochrane 1972; Warren and Mosteller 1993). The Cochrane Centre, established in Oxford by the National Health Service in 1992, is the international effort to take up Cochrane's challenge (Chalmers, Dickersin, and Chalmers 1992; Bero and Rennie 1995; McKibbon et al. 1995). It provides clinicians with information and support on clinical trials, literature searches, meta-analyses, practice guidelines, and so forth; there are eight additional affiliated Cochrane Centers in North America, Europe, and Australia, and a conceptual counterpart in the U.S. Agency for Health Care Policy and Research's program in Clinical Practice Guideline Development (Agency for Health Care Policy and Research 1993), with access available through the National Library of Medicine.

Cochrane's challenge should be understood as an ethical challenge: Bad consequences follow from uninformed decisions. Gathering data in computer databases and creating software to analyze these data are thus important tasks; they would be important even if there were no impetus to reform health care systems to reduce costs. In fact, we now have tools that allow for studying institutional outcomes in addition to aggregating data from many institutions and research studies (Safran et al. 1989).

Yet this does not solve the ethical problem whether *practice guidelines* are the best or most appropriate means to inform decision making. The problem would arise even if computers were not involved. Because they are, however, we must look at their role. (This issue will be pursued further in the discussion of meta-analysis in Chapter 8.)

Consider that one set of guidelines has been criticized because it lacks explicit definitions and specificity (Tierney et al. 1995). The conclusion here is that while computerized guidelines can represent an important synthesis of current knowledge in a field, they can be used inappropriately if they are allowed to trump decisions by individual human experts. This is not to say that the human is always right, only that a computerized guideline is one among several sources of information that clinicians should employ.

A key goal of outcomes research is to improve quality, although in some circles "quality" is a function of cost reduction and liability, not necessarily longer lives of higher quality, for instance. But one criticism of quality-of-care monitoring is that we currently have a poor understanding of risk factors, severity of illness, and complexity of care (Petryshen, Pallas, and Shamian 1995).

Moreover, mere outcomes fail to account for patient preferences and the ideal of shared decision making in clinical contexts, as is particularly evident in the case of prostate cancer and the tension between the risks of watchful waiting and surgical intervention (Wennberg, Barry, Fowler, and Mulley 1993).

Our conclusion here must therefore be the same as it was for use of prognostic scoring systems in critical care: Aggregate data, analysis, and commentary can be useful sources of evidence in clinical decision making, but we err grievously if we confuse guidelines for decision rules in individual cases. Physicians and nurses must inquire whether guidelines are consistent with their objectives and applicable to their patients (Wilson et al. 1995).

What follows from this is that, while governments, hospitals, and managed care organizations might use outcomes to compare performance and aggregate quality (Foundation for Accountability 1995; Crawford et al. 1996), it is inappropriate to require global adherence to guidelines in individual cases as a condition of employment, compensation, or evaluation. This should be uncontroversial, and understood as a celebration of the stance articulated earlier in this chapter and in Chapter 6, on use of decision-support systems.

Human subjects research

Is outcomes research a form of human subjects research? Clinical practice guidelines, algorithms, and critical pathways are based in part on analyses of previous clinical encounters. This means that data from those encounters are copied, stored, and processed for reasons that do not include the benefit of the particular patients whom the data are about. If this is research, in the sense that it is intended to produce generalizable knowledge, then by most accounts it should be subject to human subject protections.

If it is not scientific research in this sense, but, say, local "quality assessment" or the like, then perhaps it should be exempt from such review.

Suffice it to say that society must be vigilant when the distinction between patient and subject becomes blurred. When clinical information is stored in computer databases for the purpose of assessing the efficacy of interventions, it means that the circle of people and entities who claim a need to access that information has been dramatically extended.

It is generally clear and uncontroversial that no data that can be linked to particular patients should be acquired for research purposes without patient or surrogate consent (e.g., McCarthy 1991; Gold 1996). Once such data are acquired they must be accorded the same confidentiality protections as other patient data. Even if the acquisition of linked data does not subject patients to extra risks, researchers often must obtain valid consent. Such research is customarily vetted by human studies committees or institutional review boards (IRBs).

Suppose now that researchers decide to use information initially gathered for one purpose, where consent was obtained, for another purpose, for which consent would be difficult or impossible to obtain. The problem of using data for purposes other than originally intended is complex. On the one hand, using the data without consent is in conflict with one of the pillars of human subject protection. Contrarily, forgoing use of the data may constitute a missed opportunity to advance biomedical science or improve public health; too, it might be that subjects who consented to the research they knew about would also consent to future or additional analyses. What is distinctive about computer databases in such considerations is the very possibility, if not ease, of conducting the research. Once information is organized into machine-tractable databases the opportunities for research expand dramatically. (The term "machine tractable" is used to suggest about a collection of data that it has been rendered more useful and accessible to others; think of the difference between a computer disk containing dictionary entries and a networked database from which one can identify synonyms, etymology, usage examples, etc. The former is "machine readable" and the latter is "machine tractable." The term is adapted from work in natural language processing [Wilks et al. 1990].)

One way to minimize the problem of new uses for old data might be to broaden initial consent to include future studies. To be scientifically useful, however, such a move might require such vague or over-broad conditions as to be ethically meaningless. Another way to justify such (retrospective) research would be to conduct it only after all unique identifiers were decoupled from research data sets. While potentially cumbersome, such a policy is in line with the general and praiseworthy mandate to unlink patient identifiers from data and report data in aggregate. This appears to be the policy adopted by Project IMPACT, a North American effort by the Society of Critical Care Medicine to build a national database to study practice patterns, track outcomes and so forth (Society of Critical Care Medicine [no date]).

Research on health reform related issues, including outcomes, must adhere to strict confidentiality guidelines. But suppose for the sake of discussion that one wanted to conduct a retrospective study of unlinked critical care data with the goal of (1) identifying future patients from whom treatment could be withheld because of poor prognoses; (2) justifying refusals to pay or reimburse physicians for future treatments of a particular type in a specific population or prognosis group; or (3) establishing practice guidelines aimed at maximizing profits while minimizing liability (without attending to quality of care, or outcomes).

In each of these cases, an ethical issue is raised without the confidentiality of any individual patient being compromised. Nevertheless, individual patient data are being used for purposes that are inappropriate and unethical. The notion that confidentiality rights obtain only when data are coupled to unique identifiers ignores the fact that confidentiality is closely associated with the idea that individuals should generally be able to control dissemination of information about them. Unlinked data is still *about* individuals who might, if they could, object to certain uses of that data. Complicating matters is the fact that data collected for clearly less controversial uses might still be used (later or by others) for inappropriate ones.

It must be emphasized strongly that the intent here is not to assail outcomes or epidemiological research. Retrospective, surveillance, and other studies of unlinked data are vital for public health and public health policy. By the same token, epidemiology and public health are not immune to the challenge posed when data gathered for a noble purpose might later be deployed less nobly.

A related problem is that ethnic, racial, "lifestyle," professional, sexual, and other subgroups might be harmed by use or publication of unlinked data (Coughlin 1996). For instance, critical care data might be used to improve access to care by underserved populations–but it might also cause members of racial or ethnic groups to be stigmatized. Examples of such stigma followed in 1993 from initial reports that Navaho Indians were exceptionally susceptible to a form of Hantavirus (Grady 1993) and, earlier, that Haitians were a risk group for HIV and AIDS (Dickens, Gostin, and Levine 1991). A population can be harmed by research on unlinked data intended to help that population (cf. the discussion about computational epidemiology in Chapter 1).

One way to respond to such concerns is to ensure that even studies that use unlinked data be evaluated by human studies committees or institutional review boards (IRBs). Such evaluation might lead to (1) less stigmatizing study designs, (2) suggestions for appropriate reporting of results, and (3) greater sensitivity by researchers to risks to population subgroups. IRB members might be unfamiliar or uncomfortable with such issues, but given the nature of health care research this will soon be (if it isn't already) an unacceptable excuse for not providing evaluative and ethical oversight. IRB members must familiarize themselves with issues raised by health data sets and the electronic medical record (see Chapter 8). Additionally, there is much to be taught and learned about how best to balance the goals of affordable universal health care, optimized public health, and protection of human subjects, both as individuals and as members of communities.

Conclusion

We have become dependent on computers for acquiring, transmitting, storing, and processing data. We need these data to run the engines of health care delivery, guide national and global health policies, make the most of individual patient care, and maximize public health. And we are studying the potential for computers to tell us when further treatment is futile. Throughout, we operate under the well-motivated assumption that the future will be pretty much like the past: If we learn what *has* worked, we reckon we will know what *will* work. That is correct as far as it goes. We are sometimes ignorant, however, of how far that is.

The lessons for use of computers in critical care, as well as outcome tracking, guideline development, and so forth, may be summarized as follows:

- Computer-aided prognoses can help inform clinical or scientific decisions; they do not help solve problems related to ethics, values, and policy. Many such problems are not caused by lack of information or processing power.
- Disagreements about accuracy must be addressed before computational metrics are applied in patient care.
- Causation is vital to a comprehensive understanding of medical and nursing prognoses. Computer systems that do not illuminate etiology

must be handled with extreme caution, and their use delimited and perhaps constrained.

• Health care reform and cost containment are ethical imperatives that are not necessarily served by strict reliance on information processing, although they cannot ignore or forgo all information processing.

We often cannot determine in advance whether any particular decision is ethically appropriate. It is when facts are linked to values that we obtain ethical guidance. What we can do is offer standards or guidelines by which future decisions may be judged. Such standards will serve us well as we extend our use and reliance on computers in the health professions. The search for computerized algorithms to make difficult decisions easier is a strategy whose utility must not be overestimated, either in ethics or in the health professions.

References

Agency for Health Care Policy and Research. 1993. *AHCPR Program Note: Clinical Practice Guideline Development* (AHCPR Pub. No. 93–0023). Rockville, Md.: U.S. Department of Health and Human Services.

Bero, L., and Rennie, D. 1995. The Cochrane Collaboration: preparing, maintaining, and disseminating systematic reviews of the effects of health care. *Journal of the American Medical Association* 274: 1935–8.

Brody, B.A. 1989. The ethics of using ICU scoring systems in individual patient management. *Problems in Critical Care* 3: 662–70.

Castella, X., Artigas, A., Bion, J., and Kari, A. 1995. A comparison of severity of illness scoring systems for intensive care unit patients: results of a multicenter, multinational study. *Critical Care Medicine* 23: 1327–35

Castella, X., Gilabert, J., Torner, F., and Torres, C. 1991. Mortality prediction models in intensive care: Acute Physiology And Chronic Health Evaluation II and Mortality Prediction Model compared. *Critical Care Medicine* 19: 191–7.

Chalmers, I., Dickersin, K., and Chalmers, T.C. 1992. Getting to grips with Archie Cochrane's agenda. *British Medical Journal* 305: 786–8.

Civetta, J.M. 1990. New and improved scoring systems. *Critical Care Medicine* 18:1487–90.

Civetta, J.M. 1991. Scoring systems: do we need a different approach? *Critical Care Medicine* 19: 1460–1.

Civetta, J.M., Hudson-Civetta, J.A., and Nelson, L.D. 1990. Evaluation of APACHE II for cost containment and quality assurance. *Annals of Surgery* 212: 266–74.

Cochrane, A.L. 1972. *Effectiveness and Efficiency: Random Thoughts in Health Services.* London: Nuffield Provincial Hospital Trust.

Computers & Medicine. 1994. Using computer to judge care outcome is iffy. *Computers & Medicine* 23(11): 6.

Coughlin, S.C. 1996. Ethically optimized study designs in epidemiology. In

Ethics and Epidemiology, ed. S.C. Coughlin and T.L. Beauchamp, pp. 145–55. New York: Oxford University Press.

Cowen, J.S., and Kelley, M.A. 1994. Error and bias in using predictive scoring systems. *Critical Care Clinics* 10: 53–72.

Crawford, C.M., and the Health Information and Applications Working Group. 1996. Managed Care and the NII: A Public/Private Perspective (Health Care White Paper). Washington, D.C.: U.S. Department of Health and Human Services, Information Infrastructure Task Force, Committee on Applications and Technology.

Dagi, T.F. 1993. Ethics, outcomes, and epistemology: How should imprecise data figure into health-policy formulation? *Journal of Clinical Ethics* 4: 262–6.

Dickens, B.M., Gostin, L., and Levine, R.J. 1991. Research on human populations: national and international ethical guidelines. *Law, Medicine and Health Care* 19: 157–61.

Emanuel, E.J., and Emanuel, L.L. 1994. The economics of dying: the illusion of cost savings at the end of life. *New England Journal of Medicine* 330: 540–4.

Foundation for Accountability. 1995. *Guidebook for Performance Measurement.* Teton Village, Wyo.: Foundation for Accountability.

Gold, E.B. 1996. Confidentiality and privacy protection in epidemiologic research. In *Ethics and Epidemiology,* ed. S.C. Coughlin and T.L. Beauchamp, pp. 128–41. New York: Oxford University Press.

Goodman, K.W. 1996. Critical care computing: outcomes, confidentiality, and appropriate use. *Critical Care Clinics* 12:109–22.

Grady, D. 1993. Death at the corners. *Discover,* December: 82–91.

Haines, A., and Feder, G. 1992. Guidance on guidelines: Writing them is easier than making them work. *British Medical Journal* 305: 785–6.

Hippocrates. 1983. *Hippocratic Writings,* ed. G.E.R. Lloyd, trans. J. Chadwisk and W.N. Mann. London: Penguin Books.

Hume, D. 1969. *A Treatise of Human Nature,* book I, part III. Middlesex: Penguin (first published 1739 and 1740).

Iezzoni, L.I., Ash, A.S., Schwartz, M, Daley, J., Hughes, J.S., and Mackiernan, Y.D. 1995. Predicting who dies depends on how severity is measured: implications for evaluating patient outcomes. *Annals of Internal Medicine* 123: 763–70.

Jecker, N.S., and Schneiderman, L.J. 1993. Medical futility: the duty not to treat. *Cambridge Quarterly of Health Care Ethics* 2: 151–9.

Knaus, W. 1993. Ethical implications of risk stratification in the acute care setting. *Cambridge Quarterly of Healthcare Ethics* 2:193–6.

Knaus, W.A., Wagner, D.P., and Lynn, J. 1991. Short-term mortality predictions for critically ill hospitalized adults: science and ethics. *Science* 254: 389–94.

Knaus, W.A., Wagner, D.P., Draper, E.A., Zimmerman, J.E., Bergner, M., Bastos, P.G., Sirio, C.A., Murphy, D.J., Lotring, T., Damiano, A., and Harrell, F.E. 1991. The APACHE III prognostic system: risk prediction of hospital mortality for critically ill hospitalized adults. *Chest* 100: 1619–36.

Kollef, M.H., and Schuster, D.P. 1994. Predicting intensive care unit outcome with scoring systems: underlying concepts and principles. *Critical Care Clinics* 10:1–18.

Le Gall, J.R., Lemeshow, S., and Saulnier, F. 1993. A new Simplified Acute

Physiology Score (SAPS II) based on a European/North American multi-center study. *Journal of the American Medical Association* 270: 2957–63.

Lemeshow, S., Teres, D., Avrunin, J.S., and Gage, R.W. 1988. Refining intensive care unit outcome prediction by using changing probabilities of mortality. *Critical Care Medicine* 16: 470–7.

Lemeshow, S., Teres, D., Klar, J., Avrunin, J.S., Gehlbach, S.H., and Rapoport, J. 1993. Mortality Probability Models (MPM II) based on an international cohort of intensive care unit patients. *Journal of the American Medical Association* 270: 2478–86.

Luce, J.M., and Wachter, R.M. 1994. The ethical appropriateness of using prognostic scoring systems in clinical management. *Critical Care Clinics* 10: 229–41.

McCarthy, C.R. 1991. Confidentiality: the protection of personal data in epidemiological and clinical research trials. In *Ethics and Epidemiology: International Guidelines. Proceedings of the XXVth Council for International Organizations of Medical Sciences Conference,* ed. Z. Bankowski, J.H. Bryant, and J.M. Last, pp. 59–70. Geneva: CIOMS.

McKibbon, K.A., Wilczynski, N., Hayward, R.S., Walker-Dilks, C.J., and Haynes, R.B. 1995. The medical literature as a resource for health care practice. *Journal of the American Society for Information Science* 46:737–42.

Petryshen, P., Pallas, L.L.O., and Shamian, J. 1995. Outcomes monitoring: adjusting for risk factors, severity of illness, and complexity of care. *Journal of the American Medical Informatics Association* 2: 243–9.

Pollack, M.M., Ruttimann, U.E., and Getson, P.R. 1988. The pediatric risk of mortality (PRISM) score. *Critical Care Medicine* 16: 1110–16.

Rapoport, J., Teres, D., and Lemeshow, S. 1996. Resource use implications of do not resuscitate orders for intensive care unit patients. *American Journal of Respiratory and Critical Care Medicine* 153: 185–90.

Ruttimann, U.E. 1994. Statistical approaches to development and validation of predictive instruments. *Critical Care Clinics* 10:19–35.

Ruttimann, U.E., and Pollack, M.M. 1991. Objective assessment of changing mortality risks in pediatric intensive care unit patients. *Critical Care Medicine* 19: 474–83.

Safran, C., Porter, D., Lightfoot, J., Rury, C.D., Underhill, L.H., Bleich, H.L., and Slack, W.V. 1989. ClinQuery: A system for online searching of data in a teaching hospital. *Annals of Internal Medicine* 111: 751–6.

Sasse, K. 1993. Prognostic scoring systems: facing difficult decisions with objective data. *Cambridge Quarterly of Healthcare Ethics* 2: 185–91.

Schafer, J.H., Maurer, A., Jochimsen, F., Emde, C., Wegscheider, K., Arntz, H.R., Heitz, J., Krell-Schroeder, B., and Distler, A. 1990. Outcome prediction models on admission in a medical intensive care unit: do they predict individual outcome? *Critical Care Medicine* 18: 1111–18.

Schneiderman, L.J., and Jecker, N.S. 1995. *Wrong Medicine: Doctors, Patients, and Futile Treatment.* Baltimore: Johns Hopkins University Press.

Society of Critical Care Medicine. No date. Project IMPACT (brochure). Anaheim, Calif.: Society of Critical Care Medicine.

Sprung, C.L., Eidelman, L.A., and Pizov, R. 1996. Changes in forgoing life-sustaining treatments in the United States: concern for the future. *Mayo Clinic Proceedings* 71: 512–6.

Teno, J.M., Murphy, D., Lynn, J., Tosteson, A., Desbiens, N., Connors, A.F.,

Hamel, M.B., Wu, A., Phillips, R., Wenger, N., Harrell, F., and Knaus, W.A. 1994. Prognosis-based futility guidelines: Does anyone win? *Journal of the American Geriatrics Society* 42: 1202–7.

Teres, D. 1993. Trends from the United States with end of life decisions in the intensive care unit. *Intensive Care Medicine* 19: 316–22.

Teres, D., and Lemeshow, S. 1994. Why severity models should be used with caution. *Critical Care Clinics* 10: 93–110.

Tierney, W.M., Overhage, J.M., Takesue, B.Y., Harris, L.E., Murray, M.D., Vargo, D.L., and McDonald, C.J. 1995. Computerizing guidelines to improve care and patient outcomes: the example of heart failure. *Journal of the American Medical Informatics Association* 2: 316–22.

Vassar, M.J., and Holcroft, J.W. 1994. The case against using the APACHE system to predict intensive care unit outcomes in trauma patients. *Critical Care Clinics* 10: 117–26.

Warren, K.S., and Mosteller, F., eds. 1993. *Doing More Good than Harm: The Evaluation of Health Care Interventions,* Annals of the New York Academy of Sciences, vol. 703. New York: New York Academy of Sciences.

Watts, C.M., and Knaus, W.A. 1994a. The case for using objective scoring systems to predict intensive care unit outcome. *Critical Care Clinics* 10: 73–89.

Watts, C.M., and Knaus, W.A. 1994b. Comment on "Why severity models should be used with caution." *Critical Care Clinics* 10: 111–15.

Watts, C.M., and Knaus, W.A. 1994c. Comment on "The case against using the APACHE system to predict ICU outcome in trauma patients." *Critical Care Clinics* 10:129–34.

Wennberg, J.E., Barry, M.J., Fowler, F.J., and Mulley, A. 1993. Outcomes research, PORTs, and health care reform. In *Doing More Good Than Harm: The Evaluation of Health Care Interventions,* ed. K.S. Warren and F. Mosteller, Annals of the New York Academy of Sciences, vol. 703, pp. 52–62. New York: New York Academy of Sciences.

Wilks, Y., Fass, D., Guo, C., McDonald, J., Plate, T., and Slator, B. 1990. Providing machine tractable dictionary tools. *Machine Translation* 5: 99–154.

Wilson, M.C., Hayward, R.S.A., Tunis, S.R., Bass, E.B., and Guyatt, G. 1995. Users' guides to the medical literature. VII. How to use clinical practice guidelines. B. What are the recommendations and will they help you in caring for your patients? *Journal of the American Medical Association* 274: 1630–2.

Wittgenstein, L. 1968. *Philosophical Investigations,* 3rd ed., trans. G.E.M. Anscombe. Oxford: Blackwell.

Youngner, S.J. 1988. Who defines futility? *Journal of the American Medical Association* 260: 2094–5.

8

Meta-analysis: conceptual, ethical, and policy issues

KENNETH W. GOODMAN

The birth and evolution of a scientific method is an exciting development. Meta-analysis, described in this chapter as "one of the most important and controversial methodological developments in the history of science," has changed aspects of scientific inquiry in ways that have not been fully calculated. The technique is nearly as old as this century but as fresh, immediate, and important as this week's journal articles and subsequent lay accounts. In a meta-analysis, the results of previous studies are pooled and then analyzed by any of a number of statistical tools. Meta-analyses are performed on data stored in computers and subjected to computational statistics. The technique grew rapidly in psychology beginning two decades ago and since has become a fixture in the observational investigations of epidemiologists, in reviews of clinical trials in medicine, and in the other health sciences. It has engendered extraordinarily heated debate about its quality, accuracy, and appropriate applications. Meta-analysis raises ethical issues because doubts about its accuracy raise doubts about (1) the proper protections of human subjects in clinical trials; (2) the proper treatment of individual patients by their physicians, nurses, and psychologists; and (3) the correct influence on public policy debates. This chapter lays out ethical and policy issues, and argues for high educational standards for practitioners in each domain.

Introduction

The growth of knowledge presents some of the most interesting and demanding problems in all human inquiry. Questions of how we acquire beliefs about the world, how we justify them, how we determine if they are true (or whether they can be true), whether they should supplant old beliefs – these and other questions guide the efforts of epistemologists, that is, philosophers of the kinds, goals, and limits of knowledge. They

I am grateful to Professor Ed Erwin for comments on an earlier version of this paper.

also can guide the work of scientists, although with different emphasis and focus.

The history of science reveals a vast multitude of ways people have tried to learn about the world: We have looked to stars and to gods, conducted tests and experiments, and sometimes just used our heads. The question of what makes the best method for learning about natural phenomena is an especially interesting and important one in epistemology. In important respects, scientific research methods embody attempts to square data (observations, experimental results, background knowledge) with theories (or organizational lattices, matrices, or frameworks). If we see things that our theories cannot explain, we say the theories lack explanatory adequacy. Such adequacy was accepted by the ancient Greeks as the fulfillment of inquiry in cosmology: If astronomers could not learn about the *properties* of the bodies they saw, at least they could tell a coherent story about why they appeared and moved as they did. This requirement, from Plato through Eudoxus and Calippus, was that scientists should strive to "save the appearances" or "save the phenomena" (σωζειν τα φαινομενα) (Duhem 1969). This was less than truth, but it was regarded, at least in astronomy, as the best one could do.

The phenomena, or data, or observations, were the stuff that scientists tried to acquire and then to explain. To one extent or another, this stuff was of or about the world. In the modern era, in a tradition customarily traced to Bacon and Descartes, among others, scientists shake this stuff loose, tease it out, or espy it and then try to make sense of it, or use it in support of one theory or another.

In the 19th and 20th centuries the reports of scientists became data for sociologists and others. The idea that such reports could be data for anything else seems preposterous: If the scientists took their data from the world, then the only thing a scientific report itself can be data about is the activity of scientists. But this is mistaken, as any review article or survey makes plain. Customarily, a scientist who wants to learn about the lay of the land in a given domain reads an article by someone who has reviewed the published literature and gleans from it the state of knowledge in the domain: Here is what we know, suspect, want to know, and so forth. Textbooks also fill this function. The job is vast: Some 23,000 journals are published annually in the biomedical sciences; more than 8,000 new clinical trials begin each year (Olkin 1995).

Notably, survey articles constitute a comparatively unscientific way to perform such a synthesis (Mulrow 1987). Many are subjective and overlook or misinterpret important scientific evidence, especially in areas that are home to active research programs. How could it be otherwise, given the volume of research and the vastly many loci for publishing results? In fact, dissatisfaction with narrative reviews in psychology is said to have motivated the development of a more scientific review strategy (Glass and Kliegl 1983).

While there remain important reasons to commend and use the traditional survey article, there is a need for a more rigorous way of analyzing data from diverse sources – a more rigorous way of turning scientific *reports* themselves into data about the world, and then aggregating these diverse data. One such method is called "meta-analysis." This chapter identifies and evaluates methodological, conceptual, and ethical issues raised by the conduct and use of meta-analysis. Those issues include use of meta-analytic findings in subsequent clinical research and patient care, and applications of meta-analysis in formulating public policy.

Meta-analysis

The goals of research synthesis

The term "meta-analysis" was first used by a psychologist who defined it as "the statistical analysis of a large collection of results from individual studies for the purpose of integrating the findings" (Glass 1976). Since then, the idea of such systematic reviews of previous research has been applied in psychology and psychotherapy, social science, education, meteorology, marketing, management and business studies and, perhaps especially, in medicine and epidemiology, including all aspects of clinical trials, drug efficacy, disease prevention, investigator education and reporting, public health, health policy, and patient education and behavior (cf. Louis, Fineberg, and Mosteller 1985).

Meta-analysis constitutes one of the most important and controversial methodological developments in the history of science.

The idea that disparate bits or collections of information can be pooled to reveal broad-spectrum or aggregate insights is intuitively straightforward. We can think of two prime domains for such pooling. The world of natural phenomena is one. *Reports* about the world constitute the other.

Thus Glass and his colleagues defined "primary analysis" as "the original analysis of data in a research study. It is what one typically imagines as the application of statistical methods." They defined "secondary analysis" as "the reanalysis of data for the purpose of answering the original research question with better statistical techniques, or answering new questions with old data''; and ''meta-analysis'' as ''nothing more than the attitude of data analysis applied to quantitative summaries of individual experiments'' (Glass, McGaw, and Smith 1981: 21).

Examples of natural phenomena pooling include astronomers' use of a composite or Very Large Array telescope to collect information about distant phenomena, and various sampling techniques in epidemiology. By collecting signals detected across an area instead of at a point, we are able to assemble a more complete and so presumably a more accurate picture of a particular phenomenon or entity. An example of an aggregate of reports about natural phenomena can be found at any scientific meeting on a particular or restricted subject. One who attends the different presentations will gain information about several aspects of a phenomenon, and so, we suppose, assemble a more accurate picture of it. Notice that inductive inference is not necessarily involved in either example.

Of course these two examples illustrate only a small part of the large class of things we count as worthy of scientific study. In fact, most scientific inquiries are marked not by pooling of data at such a restricted level but by pooling at a wider level, or the collection of data from different or heterogeneous sources. It is from this data that we attempt to induce true statements about the class that contains the entities. In medicine, for instance, we might do a study to determine whether a particular drug prolongs life after a myocardial infarction. In such studies we administer the drug to people who have just had heart attacks and compare their survival rate to others who have had heart attacks but received either no drug or a placebo. If enough test subjects survive longer than controls, we infer that the drug is efficacious. Here we might have tens, hundreds, or thousands of entities (the test subjects) from whom we collected data over months or years. This sort of pooling is just the inductive attempt to increase knowledge about natural phenomena. Were we to look at other *studies* of the usefulness of the drug in myocardial infarctions we would be engaged in the activity of aggregating reports about the world. This is an inductive process.

There are several problems with inductions about natural phenomena. One is precisely the problem of induction itself: It is no small project to justify inferences from (1) the similarity of data about different events to (2) a causal connection between data and event-outcomes (see the discussion of induction in Chapter 7). While philosophers since Hume have identified this as a major challenge to those trying to learn about the world, it has not much bothered scientists, who tend sanguinely to understand their inductions to point to causal connections and scientific truths. A secondary problem emerges in reviews of reports. What if the reports are contradictory? That is, what if some studies lead us to induce that a particular drug is efficacious and others lead us to induce that it is not? And what if, because of small sample sizes, the reports are inconclusive?

Meta-analysis attempts in part to resolve such contradictory or inconclusive findings. As a tool for integrating or synthesizing a variety of research findings, meta-analysis attempts a sort of meta-induction. The idea is that if we take previous studies as data, we can infer from their aggregate to a causal connection that was not apparent from any individual study, or, indeed, from any cursory examination of the research record. (It has been suggested that meta-analysis can be made deductive, though this is controversial; see Maclure 1993 and the references therein.)

The literature on the method of meta-analysis is vast and extends across medicine, epidemiology, nursing, psychology, sociology, and education. A number of useful book-length treatments and collections are available (Glass, McGaw, and Smith 1981; Hedges and Olkin 1985; Wachter and Straf 1990; Cook et al. 1992; Cooper and Hedges 1994), as are several articles (Bulpitt 1988; Thacker 1988; Dickersin and Berlin 1992; Schmidt 1992; Lau and Chalmers 1995; Lau, Schmid, and Chalmers 1995; Longnecker 1995; Olkin 1995).

Historical considerations

There is nothing remarkable here so far. We have long had the idea that it is possible to make some kind of inference about natural processes and events from previous reports about the world. In some respects, this is just what we understand by saying that scientific progress is cumulative. It might be difficult to read from the published record what the accumulation adds up to, but that, we reckon, is our problem, not the record's.

The method of combining the results of several studies is often traced to an attempt at the beginning of the century to average five studies of the correlation between mortality and inoculation for typhoid fever (Pearson 1904). The average was used to estimate the effect size for typhoid inoculations and compare it with effect sizes of inoculations for other diseases. In many respects, meta-analysis remains, at core, a tool to measure and compare effect sizes. Other attempts followed in the physical and statistical sciences. Meta-analysis is in principle applicable in any science. Olkin (1990), for instance, gives a very nice example of the amalgamation of evidence from efforts in cosmology in the 1930s to determine the gravitational constant. Other significant applications emerged in agriculture (Hedges and Olkin 1985).

The quantified amalgamation of evidence progressed sporadically from the 1920s through the 1960s, consolidating in the 1970s (Olkin 1990). Work in research synthesis has burgeoned since then, driven by two important factors. The first was a vast and rapid increase in the number of studies, trials, and experiments, and the concomitant increase in the published record, especially in the health professions; the second was the development of readily accessible statistical tools and computers on which to use them.

Criticisms of meta-analysis

The meta-analyst's statistical tools are now necessarily computational. Such necessity is not logical, but practical. In principle, meta-analysis could be performed "by hand" in a way not unlike that of the first research synthesists. In fact, though, meta-analyses are performed on computers. Moreover, the statistical techniques and computational power required are not extraordinary or excessive. Meta-analysis has become a desktop enterprise.

The technique is also quite controversial – indeed, as controversial as it is popular. We can categorize criticisms of meta-analysis into two types, methodological and conceptual. Examples of the former include the problems of publication bias and research quality, including investigator bias. Examples of the latter involve the concept of a crucial experiment and the presumption of causal connections.

The criticisms are significant: A successful impeachment of meta-analytic techniques will cast doubt on claims of improved clinical care; applying a misleading meta-analysis can be dangerous. It is important to note that many methodological problems for the meta-analyst have been acknowledged and addressed by the developers and proponents of the technique (e.g., Chalmers 1991). This represents a significant trend at the intersection of ethics, computing, and medicine: From clinical decision support (Chapter 6) to prognostic severity scores (Chapter 7) to computational research synthesis, the scientists and clinicians who have been parents of the techniques have also tended to be frank in acknowledging their children's limitations and shortcomings.

Methodological issues

One of the first steps in a meta-analysis is the identification of the studies to be analyzed. This is done in several ways: citation and publication database searches by keywords, talking to colleagues, and plumbing personal knowledge of earlier research. This produces two main types of studies: published and unpublished. Published studies are well known to present the problem of publication bias, or the tendency of referees, editors, and researchers to favor publication or submission of reports with positive results, or of research supported by external funding sources (Dickersin et al. 1987; Newcombe 1987; Chalmers 1990; Dickersin 1990; Easterbrook, Berlin, Gopalan, and Matthews 1991; Dickersin, Min, and Meinert 1992; Dickersin and Min 1993a, b). A related problem is that some meta-analyses are based exclusively on reports in certain languages; one study showed that 78 percent of meta-analyses reviewed had language restrictions (Grégoire, Derderian, and Le Lorier 1995). But surely the idea of an "English-only" or "French-only" meta-analysis should be seen as problematic.

For published studies, the problem is clear: If a meta-analysis is based only on published studies it is omitting crucial data, data that might contribute to a different conclusion. Proponents of meta-analysis have responded to this by encouraging the inclusion of unpublished data, improving research quality, reducing conflicts of interest, and urging the further development of registries of such data (Simes 1986; Chalmers, Frank, and Reitman 1990); indeed, the problem of publication bias was one of the key motivations for establishing the Cochrane Collaboration (Chalmers, Dickersin, and Chalmers 1992; Warren and Mosteller 1993; Bero and Rennie 1995), the international registry of clinical trials and other data (see Chapter 7). Further, a number of tests have been proposed for identifying publication bias in meta-analyses (Begg and Mazumdar 1994), and it has been suggested that the expansion of electronic journals and other means of on-line publication will reduce publication bias (Berlin 1992).

On the other hand, one cannot conclude that most or all unpublished studies were rejected or not submitted for publication because of negative results. They might not have been published because they were poor studies, perhaps conceptually flawed or badly executed (Erwin 1984). There is no easy way of determining for any individual study the reasons it was not published. Now couple this with acknowledged shortcomings in the peer review process: Most referees spend surprisingly little time evaluating manuscripts (Lock 1990), authors of published reports often make errors in citing or quoting supporting references (Evans, Nadjari, and Burchell 1990), and referee judgments of the same submission can vary widely (Garfunkel, Ulshen, Hamrick, and Lawson 1990). The following observation becomes incontestable: If a meta-analysis is based in part on flawed reports, then the meta-analysis must in some degree be flawed also.

An important response to these criticisms is that meta-analysis itself has served to identify flawed studies that would otherwise have gone unrecognized as such. In one strong defense it is observed that "authors of meta-analyses are forever deploring poor quality in studies rather than papering it over with calculations" (Wachter 1988: 1407). This is noteworthy, but it leaves unaddressed the fact that identifying a previous study as flawed does not improve its quality for the purpose at hand.

A third problem is that meta-analyses of clinical trials do not customarily take into account data about the individual subjects on those trials, and so are aggregating unlike data. This has been called the "heterogeneity problem," or the problem of "apples and oranges" (Hunter and Schmidt 1990; Chalmers 1991; Thompson 1994). Indeed, it has been shown that different meta-analyses on the same topic will produce different results depending on whether they were based on literature synthesis, individual patient data, or unpublished trials (Jeng, Scott, and Burmeister 1995). One solution to the heterogeneity problem is to conduct more meta-analyses using individual patient data (Oxman, Clarke, and Stewart 1995), although this introduces a confidentiality challenge to data sharing, a matter to be taken up later.

Moreover, different statistical methods embody different assumptions, and this can lead to error (Thompson 1993). For instance, in a random-effects approach, it is assumed that treatment effects gleaned from individual trials are positioned randomly around a central value, thus constituting an attempt to deal with the problem of hetereogeneity; in the fixed-effects model, it is assumed that the true treatment effect is the same in each trial (Thompson and Pocock 1991).

Meta-analysis is sometimes criticized for making something out of nothing. One epidemiologist, who argues for the abandonment of meta-analyses of published observational data, writes that "meta-analysis offers the Holy Grail of attaining statistically stable estimates for effects of low magnitude" (Shapiro 1994: 771).

Another methodological criticism focuses on meta-analyses themselves and not on their input. The late Thomas Chalmers and colleagues, in a review of 86 meta-analyses of randomized controlled trials, found non-trivial shortcomings in six key areas, namely, study design, combinability, control of bias, statistical analysis, sensitivity analysis and application of results (Sacks et al. 1987; cf. Bailar 1995 for a more recent criticism of meta-analytic quality). In other words, many meta-analyses are not very good. The authors conclude:

> We believe that the best way to answer questions about the efficacy of new therapeutic or diagnostic methods is to perform well-designed randomized controlled trials of adequate size. Meta-analysis may have a role when definitive randomized trials are impossible or impractical, when randomized trials have been performed but the results are inconclusive or conflicting, or when the results of definitive studies are being awaited. Meta-analysis, like decision analysis, can give quantitative estimates of the weight of available evidence, which can be helpful in making clinical decisions. However, there is a danger that meta-analysis may be used inappropriately or indiscriminately (Sacks et al. 1987: 453).

What is apparent is that like any young technique, meta-analysis lacks a sufficient critical history, and it lacks standards (Michels 1992; Moher and Olkin 1995). We should not be surprised that the technique engenders disputes – there are still unresolved issues in the design of experiments on which meta-analyses are based, and on which clinical decisions are made.

Conceptual issues

We should look at three questions about the foundations of meta-analysis, namely, the possibility of meta-analytic confirmation, or meta-meta-analysis; the idea of meta-analyses as crucial experiments; and the problem of establishing causal connections.

Replication and confirmation. Sacks et al. (1987) and others have called for meta-analyses to be conducted like scientific experiments. While this is a sound response to the discovery of varying quality of existing meta-analyses, it is not clear how this will be possible. How, for instance, should one propose to replicate a meta-analysis? The obvious way seems to be this: Assign a team to perform a meta-analysis on a question previously subjected to meta-analytic scrutiny (cf. Landman and Dawes 1982; Erwin 1984); alternatively, two or more teams might approach the same question simultaneously.

Suppose a team is assigned the task of conducting a meta-analysis on the same question, problem, or topic as the previous meta-analysis, and the team sets out to search the literature, to identify appropriate unpublished studies, etc. If the meta-meta-analysts then produce the same or similar results as the original meta-analysts, we might be inclined to say that the initial findings have been supported or confirmed. But if the second group selected different studies, or used different statistical tools, or weighted the various studies differently, in what respect can this be counted as a confirmation? What is missing from this picture is the experimenter's ability to hold certain variables steady while changing others. A new meta-analysis cannot confirm – or for that matter falsify – another, because meta-analyses are not experiments.

Let us correct for this by stipulating that the meta-meta-analysts use the same input, same processing and statistical tools, and same weighting procedure. Now, though, any purported replication or confirmation is trivial: It would be very strange indeed if running the same computer programs on the same data produced different results! This illustrates one of the challenges of doing computational science.

None of this is to say that meta-analysis cannot be made "more scientific." It is to say that interesting conceptual issues remain to be resolved before that laurel can be conferred.

Meta-analyses as crucial experiments. The apparent beauty of randomized controlled studies of adequate size is that they seem often to produce clear or significant results about the effects of particular drugs or treatments. From this we infer that a particular hypothesis has been confirmed. Indeed, we might even understand such a study to constitute a crucial experiment, one that singularly demonstrates the truth of a hypothesis or theory. The problem is that some randomized controlled studies of the same subject either do not produce the same results or have such small sample sizes that we are wary about drawing overstrong conclusions from them. These problems are precisely what motivate many meta-analyses. What has happened over the past decade, though, is that meta-analyses have come to be seen by some as constituting crucial experiments, experiments that close the book on particular medical questions.

There are several problems with this view. Concerns about the role of auxiliary assumptions and hypotheses that arise for any experiment have yet to be addressed in terms of meta-analytic "experiments," and this renders suspect any inferences based on meta-analytic findings. Put this point a different way: We are not yet entirely clear about what assumptions are embedded in any meta-analysis. It might be, for instance, that different meta-analytic statistical packages embody different assumptions about effect sizes, sample size weights, and which research question is of interest (Normand 1995); these assumptions must muddy any attempt to infer that a particular meta-analysis has closed the book on research in a circumscribed topic.

Likewise must meta-analysts evaluate and confront the philosopher Karl Popper's argument that the Baconian, Newtonian, and Cartesian concept of an *experimentum crucis* is mistaken because there can be no confirming experiments, but only falsifying ones. What is striking here is that a meta-analysis that failed to show a positive correlation might not even be taken to be a falsification – there are just too many ways in which a meta-analysis might fail to detect a hypothesized connection, or just be wrong.

The Popperian challenge has been taken up in the context of clinical trials (Senn 1991), and it has motivated attempts to conduct deductive meta-analyses (Maclure 1993; for an opposing view, see Ng 1991). The key point here is simply that the concept of a crucial experiment is subject to much disagreement, making it unseemly to suppose that any meta-analysis can constitute one. Of course, if a meta-analysis could be a crucial experiment, it would provide a gold standard by which to measure other efforts; but it was in part the absence of a gold standard for evaluating the quality of primary research that presented a problem for evaluating meta-analyses in the first place.

Establishing causal connections. In a rare philosophical evaluation of meta-analysis, Erwin (1984) argues that the problems of integrating diverse empirical data (especially that all weighting procedures seem arbitrary) are such as to prevent proponents from claiming to have identified causal connections between psychotherapy and beneficial therapeutic outcomes. What is at issue in the other health sciences is, similarly, meta-analysis's ability to uncover such connections, or to provide evidence for the truth of universal causal hypotheses.

Identifying two events as standing in a causal relationship is as difficult as it is important, and it is very difficult indeed. Evidence that an event E caused an event E_1 usually includes data that the former preceded the latter; that the latter would not have occurred but for the former; that most times (or every time) the former occurs, the latter follows; and so on. From Aristotle through Hume and into the modern era and the rise of the philosophy of science, the problem of causation has been a core concern of those trying to understand how science can accurately describe the world. If establishing causal connections is as difficult as it is when working with primary data, whence the thesis that meta-analysis can reveal such connections? A meta-analysis is not directly about events, but about studies of events. In the absence of better warrant, a meta-analysis might strengthen a belief that there is a correlation between a drug and a cure, say, and it might even strengthen a belief that the drug caused the cure; but this is, epistemologically, very thin beer.

Erwin's conclusion for psychotherapy is that "what is needed are better theories, better taxonomies, and better empirical data" (Erwin 1984: 435). That is, meta-analysis cannot succeed where other techniques fail. This is a good lesson for the rest of health research.

Ethical issues

We can identify two broad classes of ethical issues that are raised by computational meta-analysis. One class involves human subjects research and the relation between randomized controlled trials and meta-analysis; the other involves the application of meta-analytic findings to patient care.

Meta-analysis and clinical trials

What is the proper relationship between meta-analyses and randomized controlled trials? We have so far been considering difficulties that arise for meta-analyses that are based on such trials and other human subjects research. But influence flows in the opposite direction, too. We should consider three kinds of meta-analytic influence: (1) A clinical trial is canceled or not conducted because of meta-analytic evidence; (2) a trial is modified or halted because of meta-analytic evidence; and (3) meta-analyses impedes data sharing among investigators. It is obvious that if we are concerned about the quality, data, or provenance of a meta-analysis, we should likewise be concerned about the kind and magnitude of its influence on subsequent research.

Conducting new clinical trials. Suppose a meta-analysis increases confidence in a drug treatment's efficacy. Is there any point in doing more clinical research if such research would expose subjects to risks, or cause those in a control group to miss out on an effective therapy? This question cannot be answered independently of the level of our confidence, and the degree to which we are justified in arriving at that level, based on a meta-analysis. Many critics contend that the level of confidence should be very low, and the degree very small. In other words, a meta-analysis should not generally be allowed to foreclose on future clinical research – research that might be definitive. This is a difficult ethical challenge because the failure to pursue a line of scientific inquiry can impede the development of new drugs, treatments, or procedures. The human cost of this impediment must be balanced against the risks to subjects based on uncertain or indeterminate evidence, as from meta-analyses.

Contrarily, if a meta-analysis is accurate, and we know it, it becomes unethical to expose subjects to nontrivial risk in a subsequent clinical trial. It would be inappropriate, for instance, to allow subjects to be randomized into a placebo control arm of a clinical trial if it is believed that subjects in the other arm might receive efficacious treatment. (Of course, some have argued that placebo controls are broadly unethical [Rothman and Michels 1994].)

Defenders of meta-analysis have come to regard the technique as a kind of process: In a *cumulative* meta-analysis, researchers conduct a new meta-analysis whenever a new trial on the topic of interest is published. A continuously updated meta-analysis is said to help physicians and others keep track of and "digest" a burgeoning literature (Lau et al. 1992; Henderson et al. 1995; Lau, Schmid, and Chalmers 1995). A key example of the usefulness of cumulative meta-analyses is offered in the context of the European megatrials (involving nearly 30,000 subjects) of myocardial infarction (MI) interventions. Neither of the trials (GISSI 1986; ISIS-2 1988) changed what meta-analyses purportedly revealed to be "established evidence of efficacy" of intravenous thrombolytic therapy (Lau et al. 1992; cf. Antman et al. 1992). Thousands of patients who were randomized into those trials did not receive that effective therapy.

This suggests that where a "static" meta-analysis might constitute inadequate warrant to forgo future research, a cumulative one may eliminate or reduce the need to conduct a new study with human subjects, and that such a study might be unethical. (Note that two earlier noncumulative meta-analyses reached conclusions similar to the retrospective cumulative analysis [Yusuf et al. 1985; Antiplatelet Trialists' Collaboration 1988], raising similar questions about the propriety of conducting a randomized trial.)

But the answer here will not be facile: Complicating matters somewhat, it has been noted that ISIS-2 also contributed to knowledge about subject subgroups, for instance that streptokinase was efficacious as much as 24 hours after an MI, where it had been thought that the drug must be administered much sooner to reduce mortality (this point was emphasized in 1992 by Thomas Chalmers in personal communication). A common criticism of meta-analysis is that it fails to identify such subgroup variation.

Moreover, consider the findings of an updated meta-analysis on magnesium treatment of myocardial infarctions, namely, that it is an "effective, safe, simple and inexpensive" treatment that should be broadly and immediately available (Yusuf, Koon, and Woods 1993). Those findings and hopes were dashed when a subsequent megatrial, involving nearly 60,000 subjects, refuted the meta-analysis's finding of reduced mortality from magnesium (ISIS-4 1995; Yusuf and Flather 1995). To have closed the book on intravenous magnesium after the meta-analysis, and thence to have refused on ethical grounds to enroll patients in the subsequent study, would seem now to have been major mistakes. What went wrong?

Selective identification by meta-analysts of positive studies, publication bias, analysis of studies that were too small, and inadequate sensitivity analysis have been cited as potential explanations for this "false positive meta-analysis" (Egger and Smith 1995).

The challenge can be put quite directly, as it has been by Thomas Chalmers and Joseph Lau: "When is it no longer ethical to assign patients at random to a control group in a new or definitive large trial?" (Chalmers and Lau 1993: 169). They then say that answering the question "from a statistical point of view is beyond [our] ability or training."

From an ethical point of view, however, the question will be answered as a function that ranges over risk to subjects, differences between risks of being assigned to the treatment or control groups, and expected benefits from increased knowledge (benefits that might accrue not to the subjects but to others, later). In the areas where the stakes are highest, the existing treatments most diverse, and the number of trials and meta-analyses greatest – heart attacks and cancer – these risks and benefits will be exquisitely difficult to calculate.

Such decisions can be ethically optimized in two ways. First, the idea that cumulative meta-analyses should be used in designing trials, determining their sample sizes, and evaluating data during their course is an attempt to establish a high standard of care in the field (Chalmers and Lau 1993, 1996; Henderson et al. 1995; Lau, Schmid, and Chalmers 1995). Adhering to it will give scientists, clinicians, and patients a clearer, though still flawed, sense of the upshot of all previous work. To do less, they argue, is to fail to consider salient evidence in contexts in which people might be harmed.

The second way is based on the mechanism that has evolved to protect human subjects in clinical trials, the institutional review board (IRB) or human subjects committee. Until members of such committees become familiar with meta-analysis and its strengths and limitations, there is no way to conduct a valid, case-by-case evaluation of the risks and benefits of participating in a clinical trial in a domain marked by the existence of previous trials and meta-analyses. More simply: Until IRB members learn about meta-analysis and its problems and advantages, the question whether it is ethical to enroll a person in a particular randomized controlled trial cannot adequately be answered.

That is, the higher standard of care urged for meta-analysts and investigators must be paralleled by a higher standard of care for those who evaluate human subjects research. This will be a lot of trouble and a lot of work for all concerned. There is, ethically speaking, no apparent alternative.

Stopping rules. How much evidence of a treatment's efficacy or harm is required to call a halt to an ongoing clinical trial? The question is vitally important in cases where human subjects are enrolled in trials but not receiving the optimal treatment, as for instance when subjects in the control group are receiving an alternative therapy, or a placebo. The problem of such ''stopping rules,'' or thresholds beyond which it is arguably unethical to prevent subjects from receiving the supposed best treatment, is one of the most interesting in human subjects research. The challenge is this: If a stopping rule is invoked too soon, the research is ruined and its benefits lost; if it is invoked too late, human subjects are exposed to a level of risk they never agreed to during the valid consent process (Pocock 1992; Singer 1993; Baum, Houghton, and Abrams 1994).

Meta-analyses, particularly cumulative meta-analyses, have been commended as useful mechanisms for study monitoring (Henderson et al. 1995; Begg 1996; Chalmers and Lau 1996; DerSimonian 1996; Pocock 1996). Clinical trials are overseen in part by data safety and monitoring committees (distinct from IRBs) that attempt to determine if there has been a demonstration of a treatment's effectiveness, or harm, before the formal conclusion of a study. If a treatment is shown to be better than an alternative, it becomes unethical to continue to randomize patients or keep them on protocol, and a study should be stopped.

The question whether and to what extent a meta-analysis should be used in deciding to halt a clinical trial parallels that of meta-analytic influence on decisions to commence a trial. If we take seriously the advice of cumulative meta-analysis advocates, however, and use the technique in the planning and design of a randomized control trial, then it seems unlikely there will be many cases in which a pretrial meta-analysis would lead investigators to commence the study, and a subsequent, updated analysis would lead them to halt it. The idea is just that it is unlikely that enough time will pass in which to accumulate sufficient data to overturn a sound pretrial decision, although this will obviously be less so for some long-term studies.

Further and more importantly, the conceptual and methodological problems for meta-analysis as reviewed above leave many scientists displeased at the idea that the technique should be given a large role in the momentous decision to stop a randomized controlled trial: "the amount of evidence required from a meta-analysis to establish consensus is so vaguely understood that it would be impossible to determine precise stopping rules in advance of the trial" (Begg 1996; cf. Feinstein 1996). In other words, if non-meta-analytic evidence cannot justify the invocation of a stopping rule, it is not clear how a meta-analysis can tip the balance.

Another wrinkle: Stopping rules themselves can befoul subsequent meta-analyses (Hughes, Freedman, and Pocock 1992). If a study is halted earlier than intended, it can create an artificial heterogeneity of treatment effects in later analyses. Using a meta-analysis to stop a trial thus can constitute a sort of meta-analytic cannibalism in which an analysis, instead of strengthening successors, actually poisons them.

At best, cumulative meta-analytic evidence should be included along with data from other ongoing trials in any comprehensive review of a study involving human subjects. If we regard protecting those subjects as one of the main jobs of data and safety monitoring boards, then such boards incur the burden assigned just a moment ago to institutional review boards: a better understanding of meta-analytic techniques, and how they may err.

Data sharing. It has been suggested that decisions not to conduct trials because of meta-analysis have led some researchers, who doubt the accuracy and utility of the technique, to refrain from sharing data with meta-analysts. As one biostatistician has been quoted as saying, "I know of people who have refused to put their data into a meta-analysis for just that reason – they're afraid it will close off a subject prematurely" (Mann 1990: 476).

The moral obligation of scientists to share the results of their work with others is a key component in the growth of knowledge. Science builds on itself in a variety of complex ways, and the communication of ideas is essential to progressive change. Thus the failure to share the results of inquiry has been identified as a form of research misconduct (Chalmers 1990).

That said, there are credible or potentially credible challenges to a "tell-all" policy. Reporting results prematurely, revealing certain confidential information, and disclosing some kinds of propriety commercial information can each be inappropriate. To be sure, demands for nondisclosure of commercial – or potentially commercial – data are frequently overstated (Goodman 1993), and individual cases can require close scrutiny (Fayerweather et al. 1991).

Meta-analysis relies on data sharing to a greater extent than many other scientific activities. Given the increase in use of meta-analysis and parallel concerns about the technique's accuracy, it should be clear that anything that would hinder the free flow of information is potentially blameworthy (Hogue 1991).

If it is true, as suggested just above, that a meta-analysis might have the effect of short-circuiting a valuable clinical research program, then one might try to make the case that withholding data will serve a greater good. But this is a very hard line to maintain, in part because of the difficulty in foretelling the effects of future meta-analyses. The virtues and benefits of consistency and openness generally constitute far more compelling arguments in debates over data sharing than fears of inappropriate or detrimental uses of scientific information.

Another problem: It was pointed out earlier that one solution to the heterogeneity problem is to make greater use of individual patient data in compiling meta-analyses (Oxman, Clarke, and Stewart 1995). Sharing individual patient data for research cannot be accomplished ethically unless either (1) patients provide valid consent or (2) the data are bereft of unique identifiers.

Obtaining valid consent from patients in previous or distant clinical trials can be quite difficult, if not impossible. Because the secondary research would make use of data for a purpose not originally intended, it is not generally acceptable to presume consent by the original subjects.

A better solution is to ensure that the data are not shared unless all unique identifiers have first been deleted. If the records from the original trials have been entered into databases, it should be a simple matter to use computers to delete names, addresses, national identification numbers, and the like. Human subject protections can further be ensured by submitting meta-analytic protocols using individual patient data to institutional review boards. To be sure, this presumes IRBs are competent to evaluate such protocols, but this, as has been urged, is an increasingly important requirement anyway.

Meta-analysis and patient therapy

A point that has been made in several different ways so far is this: A central problem with meta-analysis is not that it cannot in principle reveal causal connections, but that we cannot in any particular case know that it has. Causation underpins evidence. Pity thus the poor clinician *qua* epistemologist. He or she is told with increased frequency – and accuracy – that the growth of medical knowledge is so broad and rapid that only "evidence-based" approaches can distill that growth and keep the practitioner up to date (Evidence-based Medicine Working Group 1992; Sackett 1995; Taubes 1996). Meta-analysis is among the tools sought out in attempts to perform that distillation. We can eavesdrop on the debate in which meta-analysis is described as

- "Statistical alchemy" (Feinstein 1995: 71) and "statistical vigilance" (Trout 1993: 9)
- "Devoid of original thought" (Rosendaal 1994: 1325) and "the best way to utilize the information that can be obtained from clinical trials to build evidence for exemplary medical care" (Lau, Schmid, and Chalmers 1995: 56)
- "Mega-silliness" (Eysenck 1978) and a device that has "focused attention on methodological *rigor* in research reviewing" (Hedges 1990: 11, original emphasis)

Of course, health care is almost always based on one kind of evidence or another. Some of it is just false, of low quality, too late in arriving, or too complex or diverse to understand. If meta-analysis could serve as handmaiden to clinical and observational trials, helping to bring their sometimes cloudy insights into the practitioner's armamentarium, it would be a precious tool indeed.

The strong anti-meta-analysis view

Some deny that meta-analyses are of much use at all in patient care. Let us call this the "strong view." It is often articulated by emphasizing the weakness of the studies on which the analysis was crafted, or on their heterogeneity:

Conjoint or external meta-analytic monitoring will seldom, if at all, pertain to the pragmatic reality of getting results that can be directly and usefully applied for patient-care decisions. An ongoing clinical trial was presumably started for the good reason that previous trials had not suitably resolved the issue or answered the question being addressed in the current trial. If the previous trials had not provided a pertinent answer before, however, they cannot suddenly become pertinent when transmogrified with meta-analytic mathematics'' (Feinstein 1996: 1279–80).

Such robust skepticism invites the following rejoinder: No one intends to make poor, inaccurate, or irrational decisions in patient care. The problem faced by practitioners is how to identify and synthesize the vast and sometimes contradictory volume of information on which sound clinical decisions are made. Unfortunately, many physicians, nurses, psychologists, and others muddle through the hard cases whether there has been meta-analytic review or not.

The question that should be asked is, "Should a meta-analysis be allowed to increase the warrant for a belief, or must the method always be disdained?" On the strong view, the answer is that meta-analysis adds nothing that was not known before, and so should carry no weight in individual treatment decisions. This position sets very high confidence levels in justifying the application of meta-analytic findings. On the strong view the term "findings" would be unacceptable.

A modified strong view might place a higher burden on those who would use a meta-analysis in individual patient decisions. That is, we might insist that no method be applied in patient care unless its advantages and disadvantages are (somewhat) familiar to practitioners. We may surmise that, despite the ubiquity of meta-analytic reports in the medical, nursing, psychological, and social science literature, most practitioners are innocent of the controversy that surrounds the method, as well as its statistical underpinnings. (A survey of physicians' or nurses' familiarity with meta-analysis would be an interesting research project in itself.) Then we would say not that meta-analysis must always be disdained, but that one must understand it before applying it. As it is, we do not know how extensively meta-analysis results are applied or relied on.

The strong view has the advantage of dissuading clinicians from placing too much weight on a meta-analysis, but it does this at the expense of not allowing them to place any weight on it.

The provisional meta-analytic view

There is a lot wrong with meta-analysis: Exemplars are based on diverse data, sometimes sloppily collected; the method fails to reveal causal connections; and it is not always practiced or reported under high standards. Still, it has evolved and been challenged in ways that have improved it. The evolution of clinical trial repositories is an important response to criticisms of publication bias and a lack of comprehensiveness. Some meta-analyses seem to produce false positives, but others parallel conclusions drawn by traditional methods. This suggests an opportunity for a modified view, or one that provisionally accepts certain meta-analytic results in the absence of more robust support for individual decisions.

In this view, a meta-analysis cannot trump other (clinical, observational, trial-based) evidence. Rather, it becomes one of several devices in the practitioner's tool kit: "Meta-analysis cannot tell clinicians how to treat an individual patient but it can provide information that helps decision making (Thompson and Pocock 1991). This parallels what has been called the "standard view" concerning use of decision-support systems in clinical medicine (Miller 1990; see also the discussion in Chapter 6; further, note the postulation in Chapter 7 of a "standard theory" on use of prognostic scoring systems in critical care).

This view acknowledges that evidentiary warrant for scientific beliefs is diverse and rarely, if at all, unitary. Hopes that meta-analysis – or any method, for that matter – will make difficult decisions into easy ones are misleading and inappropriate. The ability to sift and weigh evidence, to apply critical thought to real-world problems, is one of the most fundamental (and undertaught) skills in health care. Neither meta-analysis nor any other technique provides magic bullets (or guns, firing ranges, or armament factories!) for clinical decision making.

What remains is the need for guidance on how to weigh meta-analytic and other evidence. This is perhaps the greatest challenge for practitioners:

Probably the most important caveat in interpreting meta-analytic results is that the findings must be considered primarily hypothesis-generating rather than hypothesis-testing. Strong recommendations for treatment should not be made on the basis of even the most promising meta-analysis in the absence of a sufficiently large and well-designed trial. At the same time, data from large trials are not necessarily definitive for patients who do not fit inclusion criteria or for drug regimens that differ importantly in dose, route, or administration" (Borzak and Ridker 1995: 876; cf. Sacks et al. 1987 and Boissel et al.1989).

There is an ethical imperative here, and it is this: The scientific foundations of clinical practice impose heavy burdens on practitioners. These burdens include adequate education and continuing education in the very methods that inform clinical practice. To fail to have some grasp of how biologists, epidemiologists, clinical trialists, and others learn about humans and their maladies is to slip beneath a standard of care that helps protect patients. Medical ''cookbooks,'' algorithms, and practice guidelines are poor substitutes for *understanding*. This is not to say that guidelines are not useful; it is to say they are insufficient.

This point echoes that made above for members of institutional review boards, and it captures the insight just identified for the ''modified strong view,'' namely, that for meta-analysis and any other attempt to learn about the world, one must understand the method before applying it. This ethical requirement alone may prevent many practitioners from making too much of computational research synthesis.

Meta-analysis and public policy

In addition to medical and psychological treatments, meta-analysis is used to aggregate data from studies with immediate implications for social policy. From school desegregation (Ingram 1990) and juvenile delinquency (Lipsey 1992) to the role of nurses in health care (Brown and Grimes 1993) and the effects of living near high-voltage power lines (Washburn et al. 1994), meta-analysis has been aimed at a variety of difficult and controversial issues (Mann 1994). Indeed, this might represent the world's most unrecognized use of computing to influence public policy.

We should linger briefly at a controversial health policy issue that has been addressed by meta-analysis and see if the stance taken so far is applicable in the realm of public policy.

Environmental tobacco smoke

In January 1993 the United States Environmental Protection Agency (EPA) released a report classifying environmental or ''second-hand'' tobacco smoke as a Group A carcinogen, a category that includes radon, asbestos, and benzene, and that is reserved for the most dangerous human carcinogens (Environmental Protection Agency 1993). The report was based on a meta-analysis of 11 U.S. studies of smokers' spouses, and excluded a number of studies done outside the United States.

The report has been a source of no small controversy since then. That it contained a meta-analysis at its core has heightened debate. Misunderstandings and purported misunderstandings of meta-analysis have given us an important case at the intersection of meta-analysis and public policy, with a dollop of journalistic responsibility thrown in (Sullum 1994). The key question, of course, is, "Should and to what extent should meta-analysis be used in crafting public policy?" Certainly it will break few compassionate hearts if the effect of a meta-analysis is to reduce the exposure of children, say, to tobacco smoke. But consider the following remark, reported by Feinstein (1992): "Yes, it's rotten science, but it's in a worthy cause. It will help us to get rid of cigarettes and to become a smoke-free society."

Put thus, the idea that research believed to be flawed might nonetheless influence policy is offensive, no matter what the intentions of the policy makers might be (cf. Gori 1994; Jinot and Bayard 1994). In one respect, the very idea is incoherent: If one believes the science to be flawed, then how can it support a worthy cause? How even can the cause become worthy in the absence of credible evidence? (If environmental smoke does not harm children then there is no reason to protect them from it, and so protecting them cannot be worthy.) But granting for the sake of discussion that the cause is worthy, it is nevertheless a severe form of ethical shortsightedness to suggest that the credibility of scientists, government institutions, and policy makers is a fair trade for a victory on one policy issue. Even the most craven utilitarian would recognize this to be a bad bet.

The debate over second-hand tobacco smoke has produced a secondary literature and further refinements and criticisms of the original EPA data (e.g., Bero, Glantz, and Rennie 1994). What we are left with is familiar doubt about the upshot of a meta-analysis. The denouement should not surprise: A meta-analysis with policy implications, like any other scientific method or report, should be subjected to rigorous scrutiny, and be considered as one datum among many by policy makers. Indeed, if journalists are going to report on meta-analyses from the scientific literature, they, too, have an ethical obligation to know at least a little of what they are writing or broadcasting about. Controversy is good, but uninformed controversy is hollow and fatuous.

In this respect, public policy, like research and clinical practice, is best served by more and better science, and by participants who have an understanding of the tools of the trade, especially the new tools, and their reliance on computers.

Conclusion

It is often difficult to separate conceptual and methodological issues from ethical ones. The latter are shaped by the former. To the degree that we are unsure of any research technique's accuracy, we must confront the problem of when, if ever, it is appropriate to apply its findings to patient care, research protocols, or public policy.

Because the technique is so young, so potentially fruitful, and so open to criticisms that touch its conceptual core, meta-analysis must be handled with care. While meta-analysis can give a sort of inductive support to certain scientific hypotheses, one must exercise the greatest caution in making decisions based on its results. We might be warranted in allowing meta-analysis to contribute to our epistemic confidence, but meta-analysis should not single-handedly establish a scientific or clinical belief. (In the absence of any such belief, perhaps because existing clinical studies are few and individually inconclusive, and in case some sort of decision must be made, meta-analytic findings may be applied. But this is clearly a temporary and stop-gap measure.)

The need to take great care will increase as databases of clinical trials are developed, as meta-analysis spreads to genomics, particularly of stigmatizing diseases (Morton 1995; Shaikh et al. 1996), and as the power of desktop computing increases. Meta-analysis will become more decentralized and available to anyone who wants to use a computer to integrate data from a variety of sources. Confidence that comes from having computers give us answers to scientific questions must be tempered with restraint shaped by those experiences in which we were so enthralled by the medium that we got the wrong message.

References

Antiplatelet Trialists' Collaboration. 1988. Secondary prevention of vascular disease by prolonged antiplatelet treatment. *British Medical Journal* 296: 320–31.

Antman, E.M., Lau, J., Kupelnick, B., Mosteller, F., and Chalmers, T.C. 1992. A comparison of results of meta-analyses of randomized control trials and recommendations of clinical experts. *Journal of the American Medical Association* 268: 240–8.

Bailar, J.C. 1995. The practice of meta-analysis. *Journal of Clinical Epidemiology* 48: 149–57.

Baum, M., Houghton, J., and Abrams, K. 1994. Early stopping rules – clinical perspectives and ethical considerations. *Statistics in Medicine* 13: 1459–69.

Begg, C.B. 1996. The role of meta-analysis in monitoring clinical trials. *Statistics in Medicine* 15: 1299–1306.

Begg, C.B., and Mazumdar, M. 1994. Operating characteristics of a rank correlation test for publication bias. *Biometrics* 50: 1088–101.

Berlin, J.A. 1992. Will publication bias vanish in the age of online journals?
Online Journal of Current Clinical Trials, July 8: Document No. 12.

Bero, L., and Rennie, D. 1995. The Cochrane Collaboration: preparing, maintaining, and disseminating systematic reviews of the effects of health care.
Journal of the American Medical Association 274: 1935–8.

Bero, L.A., Glantz, S.A., and Rennie, D. 1994. Publication bias and public
health policy on environmental tobacco smoke. *Journal of the American
Medical Association* 272: 133–6.

Boissel, J.-P., Blanchard, J., Panak, E., Payrieux, J.-C., and Sacks, H. 1989.
Considerations for the meta-analysis of randomized clinical trials: summary
of a panel discussion. *Controlled Clinical Trials* 10: 254–81.

Borzak, S., and Ridker, P.M. 1995. Discordance between meta-analyses and
large-scale randomized, controlled trials: examples from the management of
acute myocardial infarction. *Annals of Internal Medicine* 123: 873–7.

Brown, S.A., and Grimes, D.E. 1993. *Nurse Practitioners and Certified Nurse-
Midwives: A Meta-Analysis of Studies on Nurses in Primary Care Roles.*
Washington, D.C.: American Nurses Publishing.

Bulpitt, C.J. 1988. Meta-analysis. *Lancet* ii: 93–4.

Chalmers, I. 1990. Underreporting research is scientific misconduct. *Journal of
the American Medical Association* 263: 1405–8.

Chalmers, I., Dickersin, K., and Chalmers, T.C. 1992. Getting to grips with Archie Cochrane's agenda. *British Medical Journal* 305: 786–8.

Chalmers, T.C. 1991. Problems induced by meta-analyses. *Statistics in Medicine*
10: 971–80.

Chalmers, T.C., Frank, C.S., and Reitman, D. 1990. Minimizing the three stages
of publication bias. *Journal of the American Medical Association* 263: 1392–
5.

Chalmers, T.C., and Lau, J. 1993. Meta-analytic stimulus for changes in clinical
trials. *Statistical Methods in Medical Research* 2: 161–72.

Chalmers, T.C., and Lau, J. 1996. Changes in clinical trials mandated by the
advent of meta-analysis. *Statistics in Medicine* 15: 1263–8.

Cook, T.D., Cooper, H., Cordray, D.S., Hartman, H., Hedges, L.V., Light, R.J.,
Louis, T.A., and Mosteller, F., eds. 1992. *Meta-Analysis for Explanation: A
Casebook.* New York: Russell Sage Foundation.

Cooper, H., and Hedges, L.V., eds. 1994. *The Handbook of Research Synthesis.*
New York: Russell Sage Foundation.

DerSimonian, R. 1996. Meta-analysis in the design and monitoring of clinical
trials. *Statistics in Medicine* 15: 1237–48.

Dickersin, K. 1990. The existence of publication bias and risk factors for its oc-
currence. *Journal of the American Medical Association* 263: 1385–9.

Dickersin, K., and Berlin, J.A. 1992. Meta-analysis: state of the science. *Epidemiologic Reviews* 14: 154–76.

Dickersin, K., and Min, Y.I. 1993a. Publication bias: the problem that won't go
away. In *Doing More Good Than Harm: The Evaluation of Health Care
Interventions,* ed. K.W. Wachter and F. Mosteller, Annals of the New York
Academy of Sciences, vol. 703, pp. 135–46. New York: New York Academy of Sciences.

Dickersin, K., and Min, Y.I. 1993b. NIH clinical trials and publication bias. *On-
line Journal of Current Clinical Trials,* April 28: Document No. 50.

Dickersin, K., Min, Y.-I., and Meinert, C.L. 1992. Factors influencing publication of research results: follow-up of applications submitted to two institutional review boards. *Journal of the American Medical Association* 267: 374–8.

Dickersin, K., Chan, S., Chalmers, T.C., Sacks, H.S., and Smith, H. 1987. Publication bias and clinical trials. *Controlled Clinical Trials* 8: 343–53.

Duhem, P. 1969. *To Save the Phenomena: An Essay on the Idea of Physical Theory from Plato to Galileo*, trans. E. Dolan and C. Maschler. Chicago: University of Chicago Press.

Easterbrook, P.J., Berlin, J.A., Gopalan, R., and Matthews, D.R. 1991. Publication bias in clinical research. *Lancet* 337: 867–72.

Egger, M., and Smith, G.D. 1995. Misleading meta-analysis: lessons from "an effective, safe, simple" intervention that wasn't. *British Medical Journal* 310: 752–4.

Environmental Protection Agency. 1993. *Respiratory Health Effects of Passive Smoking: Lung Cancer and Other Disorders.* Washington, D.C.: Government Printing Office (EPA/600/6–90/006F; GPO: 0555–000–00407–2).

Erwin, E. 1984. Establishing causal connections: meta-analysis and psychotherapy. *Midwest Studies in Philosophy* 9: 421–36.

Evans, J.T., Nadjari, H.I., and Burchell, S.A. 1990. Quotational and reference accuracy in surgical journals. *Journal of the American Medical Association* 263: 1353–4.

Evidence-based Medicine Working Group. 1992. Evidence-based medicine: a new approach to teaching the practice of medicine. *Journal of the American Medical Association* 268: 2420–5.

Eysenck, H.J. 1978. An exercise in mega-silliness. *American Psychologist* 33: 517.

Fayerweather, W.E., Tirey, S.L., Baldwin, J.K., and Hoover, B.K. 1991. Issues in data sharing and access: an industry perspective. *Journal of Occupational Medicine* 33: 1253–6.

Feinstein, A.R. 1992. Critique of review article, "Environmental tobacco smoke: Current assessment and future directions." *Toxicologic Pathology* 20: 303–5.

Feinstein, A.R. 1995. Meta-analysis: statistical alchemy for the 21st century. *Journal of Clinical Epidemiology* 48: 71–9.

Feinstein, A.R. 1996. Meta-analysis and meta-analytic monitoring of clinical trials. *Statistics in Medicine* 15: 1273–80.

Garfunkel, J.M., Ulshen, M.H., Hamrick, H.J., and Lawson, E.E.. 1990. Problems identified by second review of accepted manuscripts. *Journal of the American Medical Association* 263: 1369–71.

GISSI (Gruppo Italiano per lo Studio della Streptochinasi nell'Infarto Miocardico). 1986. Effectiveness of intravenous thrombolytic treatment in acute myocardial infarction. *Lancet* i: 397–402.

Glass, G.V. 1976. Primary, secondary, and meta-analysis of research. *Educational Researcher* 5: 3–8.

Glass, G., and Kliegl, R. 1983. An apology for research integration in the study of psychotherapy. *Journal of Consulting and Clinical Psychology* 51: 28–41.

Glass, G.V., McGaw, B., and Smith, M.L. 1981. *Meta-Analysis in Social Research.* Newbury Park, Calif.: Sage Publications.

Goodman, K.W. 1993. Intellectual property and control. *Academic Medicine* 68 (Suppl. 1): S88–S91.

Gori, G.B. 1994. Science, policy, and ethics: the case of environmental tobacco smoke. *Journal of Clinical Epidemiology* 47: 325–34.

Grégoire, G., Derderian, F., and Le Lorier, J. 1995. Selecting the language of the publications included in a meta-analysis: Is there a Tower of Babel bias? *Journal of Clinical Epidemiology* 48: 159–63.

Hedges, L.V. 1990. Directions for future methodology. In *The Future of Meta-Analysis,* ed. K.W. Wachter and M.L. Straf, pp. 11–26. New York: Russell Sage Foundation.

Hedges, L.V., and Olkin, I. 1985. *Statistical Methods for Meta-Analysis.* San Diego: Academic Press.

Henderson, W.G., Moritz, T., Goldman, S., Copeland, J., and Sethi, G. 1995. Use of cumulative meta-analysis in the design, monitoring, and final analysis of a clinical trial: a case study. *Controlled Clinical Trials* 16: 331–41.

Hogue, C.J.R. 1991. Ethical issues in sharing epidemiologic data. *Journal of Clinical Epidemiology* 44 (Suppl. 1): 103S-7S.

Hughes, M.D., Freedman, L.S., and Pocock, S.J. 1992. The impact of stopping rules on heterogeneity of results in overviews of clinical trials. *Biometrics* 48: 41–53.

Hunter, J.E., and F.L. Schmidt. 1990. *Methods of Meta-Analysis: Correcting Error and Bias in Research Findings.* New York: Sage.

Ingram, L. 1990. An overview of the desegregation meta-analyses. In *The Future of Meta-Analysis,* ed. K.W. Wachter and M.L. Straf, pp. 61–70. New York: Russell Sage Foundation.

ISIS-2 (Second International Study of Infarct Survival) Collaborative Group. 1988. Randomised trial of intravenous streptokinase, oral aspirin, both, or neither among 17,187 cases of suspected acute myocardial infarctions. *Lancet* ii: 349–60.

ISIS-4 (Fourth International Study of Infarct Survival) Collaborative Group. 1995. ISIS-4: a randomised factorial trial assessing early oral captopril, oral mononitrite, and intravenous magnesium sulfatein 58,050 patients with suspected acute myocardial infarction. *Lancet* 345: 669–85.

Jeng, G.T., Scott, J.R., and Burmeister, L.F. 1995. A comparison of meta-analytic results using literature vs individual patient data. *Journal of the American Medical Association* 274: 830–6.

Jinot, J., and Bayard, S. 1994. Respiratory health effects of passive smoking: EPA's weight-of-evidence analysis. *Journal of Clinical Epidemiology* 47: 339–49.

Landman, J., and Dawes, R. 1982. Psychotherapy outcome: Smith and Glass' conclusions stand up under scrutiny. *American Psychologist* 37: 504–16.

Lau, J., Antman, E.M., Jimenez-Silva, J., Kupelnick, B., Mosteller, F., and Chalmers, T.C. 1992. Cumulative meta-analysis of therapeutic trials for myocardial infarction. *New England Journal of Medicine* 327: 248–54.

Lau, J., and Chalmers, T.C. 1995. The rational use of drugs in the 21st century: important lessons from cumulative meta-analyses of randomized control trials. *International Journal of Technology Assessment in Health Care* 11: 509–22.

Lau, J., Schmid, C.H., and Chalmers, T.C. 1995. Cumulative meta-analysis of clinical trials builds evidence for exemplary medical care. *Journal of Clinical Epidemiology* 48: 45–57.

Lipsey, M.W. 1992. Juvenile delinquency treatment: a meta-analytic inquiry into the variability of effects. In *Meta-Analysis for Explanation: A Casebook,* ed., T.D. Cook, H. Cooper, D.S. Cordray, H. Hartman, L.V. Hedges, R.J.

Light, T.A. Louis, and F. Mosteller, pp. 83–127. New York: Russell Sage Foundation.

Lock, S. 1990. What do peer reviewers do? *Journal of the American Medical Association* 263: 1341–3.

Longnecker, M.P. 1995. Meta-analysis. In *Tools for Evaluating Health Technologies: Five Background Papers*, U.S. Congress, Office of Technology Assessment, BP-H-142. Washington, D.C.: U.S. Government Printing Office, pp. 93–123.

Louis, T.A., Fineberg, H.V., and Mosteller, F. 1985. Findings for public health from meta-analyses. *Annual Review of Public Health.* 6: 1–20.

Maclure, M. 1993. Demonstration of deductive meta-analysis: ethanol intake and risk of myocardial infarction. *Epidemiologic Reviews* 15: 328–51.

Mann, C.C. 1990. Meta-analysis in the breech. *Science* 249: 476–80.

Mann, C.C. 1994. Can meta-analysis make policy? *Science* 266: 960–2.

Michels, K.B. 1992. Quo vadis meta-analysis? A potentially dangerous tool if used without adequate rules. In *Important Advances in Oncology*, ed. V.T. DeVita, S. Hellman, and S.A. Rosenberg, pp. 243–8. Philadelphia: Lippincott.

Miller, R.A. 1990. Why the standard view is standard: people, not machines, understand patients' problems. *Journal of Medicine and Philosophy* 15: 581–91.

Moher, D., and Olkin, I. 1995. Meta-analysis of randomized controlled trials: a concern for standards. *Journal of the American Medical Association* 274: 1962–3.

Morton, N.E. 1995. Meta-analysis in complex diseases. *Clinical and Experimental Allergy* 25 (Suppl. 2): 110–12.

Mulrow, C.D. 1987. The medical review article: state of the science. *Annals of Internal Medicine* 106: 485–8.

Newcombe, R.G. 1987. Towards a reduction in publication bias. *British Medical Journal* 295: 656–9.

Ng, S.K. 1991. Does epidemiology need a new philosophy? A case study of logical inquiry in the acquired immunodeficiency syndrome epidemic. *American Journal of Epidemiology* 133: 1073–7.

Normand, S.-L.T. 1995. Meta-analysis software: a comparative review. *American Statistician* 49: 298–309.

Olkin, I. 1990. History and goals. In *The Future of Meta-Analysis*, ed. K.W. Wachter and M.L. Straf, pp. 3–10. New York: Russell Sage Foundation.

Olkin, I. 1995. Meta-analysis: reconciling the results of independent studies. *Statistics in Medicine* 14: 457–72.

Oxman, A.D., Clarke, M.J., and Stewart, L.A. 1995. From science to practice: meta-analyses using individual patient data are needed. *Journal of the American Medical Association* 274: 845–6.

Pocock, S.J. 1992. When to stop a clinical trial? *British Medical Journal* 305: 235–40.

Pocock, S.J. 1996. The role of external evidence in data monitoring of a clinical trial. *Statistics in Medicine* 15: 1285–93.

Pearson, K. 1904. Report on certain enteric fever inoculation statistics. *British Medical Journal* 2: 1243–6.

Rosendaal, F.R. 1994. The emergence of a new species: the professional meta-analyst. *Journal of Clinical Epidemiology* 47: 1325–6.

Rothman, K.J., and Michels, K.B. 1994. The continuing unethical use of placebo controls. *New England Journal of Medicine* 331: 394–8.

Sackett, D.L. 1995. Applying overviews and meta-analysis at the bedside. *Journal of Clinical Epidemiology* 48: 61–6.

Sacks, H.S., Berrier, J., Reitman, D., Ancona-Berk, V.A., and Chalmers, T.C. 1987. Meta-analyses of randomized controlled trials. *New England Journal of Medicine* 316: 450–5.

Schmidt, F.L. 1992. What do data really mean? Research findings, meta-analysis, and cumulative knowledge in psychology. *American Psychologist* 47: 1173–81.

Senn, S.J. 1991. Falsificationism and clinical trials. *Statistics in Medicine* 10: 1679–92.

Shaikh, S., Collier, D.A., Sham, P.C., Ball, D., Aitchison, K., Vallada, H., Smith, I., Gill, M., and Kerwin, R.W. 1996. Allelic association between a Ser-9-Gly polymorphism in the dopamine D3 receptor gene and schizophrenia. *Human Genetics* 97: 714–19.

Shapiro, S. 1994. Meta-analysis/shmeta-analysis. *American Journal of Epidemiology* 140: 771–8.

Simes, R.J. 1986. Publication bias: the case for an international registry of clinical trials. *Journal of Clinical Oncology* 4: 1529–41.

Singer, D.E. 1993. Problems with stopping rules in trials of risky therapies: the case of warfarin to prevent stroke in atrial fibrillation. *Clinical Research* 41: 482–6.

Sullum, J. 1994. Passive reporting on passive smoke. *Media Critic* 1(4): 41–7.

Taubes, G. 1996. Looking for the evidence in medicine. *Science* 272: 22–4.

Thompson, S.G. 1993. Controversies in meta-analysis: the case of the trials of serum cholesterol reduction. *Statistical Methods in Medical Research* 2: 173–92.

Thompson, S.G. 1994. Why sources of heterogeneity in meta-analysis should be investigated. *British Medical Journal* 309: 1351–5.

Thompson, S.G., and Pocock, S.J. 1991. Can meta-analysis be trusted? *Lancet* 338:1127–30.

Thacker, S.B. 1988. Meta-analysis: a quantitative approach to research integration. *Journal of the American Medical Association* 259: 1685–9.

Trout, J.D. 1993. Robustness and integrative survival in significance testing: the world's contribution to rationality. *British Journal for the Philosophy of Science* 44: 1–15.

Wachter, K.W. 1988. Disturbed by meta-analysis? *Science* 241: 1407–8.

Wachter, K.W., and Straf, M.L., eds. 1990. *The Future of Meta-Analysis.* New York: Russell Sage Foundation.

Warren, K.S., and Mosteller, F., eds. 1993. *Doing More Good Than Harm: The Evaluation of Health Care Interventions,* Annals of the New York Academy of Sciences, vol. 703. New York: New York Academy of Sciences.

Washburn, E.P., Orza, M.J., Berlin, J.A., Nicholson, W.J., Todd, A.C., Frumkin, H., and Chalmers, T.C. 1994. Residential proximity to electricity transmission and distribution equipment and risk of childhood leukemia, childhood lymphoma, and childhood nervous system tumors; systematic review, evaluation, and meta-analysis. *Cancer Causes and Control* 5: 299–309.

Yusuf, S., Collins, R., Peto, R., Furberg, C., Stempfer, M.J., Goldhaber, S.Z., et al. 1985. Intravenous and intracoronary fibrinolytic therapy in acute myocardial infarction: overview of results on mortality, reinfarction and side-effects from 33 randomized controlled trials. *European Heart Journal* 6: 556–85.

Yusuf, S., and Flather, M. 1995. Magnesium in acute myocardial infarction: ISIS 4 provides no grounds for its routine use. *British Medical Journal* 310: 751–2.

Yusuf, S., Koon, T., and Woods, K. 1993. Intravenous magnesium in acute myocardial infarction: an effective, safe, simple, and inexpensive intervention. *Circulation* 87: 2043–6

Index